SCC
$25.30

COMPLETE REVIEW GUIDE
For State & National Examinations In Therapeutic Massage & Bodywork

INTRODUCTION

This book is designed to provide, in a concise format, the majority of information needed to complete a successful **review** of the material tested by many states, and NCBTMB. Every effort has been made to ensure the accuracy of information contained herein. On page iii is a section entitled "Tips For Successful Test Taking." On page vi is a section entitled "Content Outline." Sample questions are provided at the end of each section to test comprehension and retention of the material presented. An answer key is found at the end of the text.

This book is not intended to be used as a primary text for the study of the disciplines covered. A listing of **Works Cited** is provided in this text, and a reference list is also included by the NCBTMB in their candidate handbook (800-296-0664 or www.ncbtmb.com).

Check with individual states for the pertinent information regarding their laws and statutes.

Using the table of contents found on page xv, one can quickly identify any areas of special interest. It is recommended that you systematically work through the text, noting in the margins any areas for further study. The **Works Cited** section provides additional resources for detailed information on specific subjects.

5th Edition - 2005   **ISBN 0-9711926-4-2   Copyright - Pine Island Publishers, Inc.**
                         ISBN 978-0-9711926-4-5
4th Edition - 2002   **ISBN 0-9711926-0-X**
3rd Edition - 1997
2nd Edition - 1996
1st Edition - 1995

For information on this and other publications please contact:

Pine Island Publishers, Inc.   **www.PineIslandPublishers.com**
800-400-1892   **www.ExamReviews.com**

D1411351

ACKNOWLEDGMENTS

Greatest appreciation to everyone who had a part in this on-going endeavor.
Special thanks to:

Leigh L. Reynolds, B.E.E., Dipl OM, L Ac.:
For her contributions to the Non-Western
Anatomy & TCM sections, advice, and continuing support.

Kay Hugghins, JD:
For her copy-editing and support.

Christine J. Heffner, R.D.H., L.M.T.:
For her countless hours at the computer &
For transforming my original notes into a coherent rendering.

James W. Megonnell, A.A.:
For lending his production expertise and PC skill.

Bridget Welch, B.S., L.M.T.:
For her editorial and organizational skills.

Christine Reuter,
For the cover layout and design.

All my students, teachers, and colleagues who continue to educate me.

ABOUT THE AUTHOR

Dr. Patrick Barron earned his Bachelor's and Master's Degrees in Rehabilitation from Marshall University in Huntington, WV and his medical degree from Bastyr University in Seattle, WA. He completed two years post-doctoral training at the University of Washington. Dr. Barron holds a medical license in the state of Washington and is a licensed massage therapist. He has been in private practice, specializing in physical medicine and rehabilitation since 1984 and is Director of Oviedo Physical Medicine, a medical and educational consulting group. He has for over 20 years been an instructor of Anatomy & Physiology, Pathology, Hydrotherapy, and various medical sciences. Dr. Barron is the founder of the Central Florida School of Health Sciences and currently teaches at several colleges in Florida.

TIPS FOR SUCCESSFUL TEST TAKING

Included below are strategies for learning, coping with test anxiety, and conquering the multiple-choice test. Basically, we want to help you to be smarter than the test you take. By making an earnest effort to complete a few basic strategic exercises, you can realize your goals. These tried and true methods require only your participation and diligence to ensure test-taking success.

PLANNING:

1. Make A Study Plan

    a. Set a time frame (and projected date) for taking your test
    b. Get the "correct" information about your test
    c. Get all test materials: application, notes, review materials, tapes, etc.
    d. Follow your test-preparation schedule

    For example:
- 10 to 12 weeks before test date - request all application materials
- 8 weeks before test - set aside 1 hr /day for review (5 days/wk)
- 4 to 6 weeks before test - confirm test date, test location, continue to review (4 days/wk) & take sample test 3 times /wk, meet with your study group once each week
- 1 to 2 weeks before test - take 2 more sample tests, focus on being well rested and relaxed about your test
- Day of test - wake early, eat a normal breakfast, allow adequate time for travel, and arrive at test site with enough time to relax & breath

2. Carry Out Your Study Plan

    a. Find a quiet spot with good light and turn OFF the stereo and TV
If you must have music, be very selective - Baroque Music has shown promise in facilitating learning. (remember, there will be no music playing when you take the test)
    b. Consider studying with others - There are both pros and cons to study groups: (group members can reinforce, clarify & support, but may also distract)
    c. Plan your study time - Determine the times that are available to you and those times at which you are most alert. Does exercise, food, coffee, etc. energize or fatigue you?
    d. Stick to your plan - Write down your schedule, don't let yourself get discouraged, reorganize your schedule and materials as necessary

LEARNING STRATEGIES:

1. **Learning styles** - How do you learn?

   a. Visual learners comprehend and retain best when they SEE the material
   b. Auditory learners comprehend and retain best when they HEAR the material
   c. Kinesthetic learners comprehend and retain best when they TOUCH (write, draw, or diagram) the material

   ### Take advantage of your learning strengths!

   Depending on your personal learning style, you may learn more efficiently by either:
   a. Annotating - Underlining or highlighting. Remember! Highlight only the main ideas of the text.
   b. Outlining - List the "Main Ideas" of text followed by the "Major details" which are then followed by the "Minor details"
   c. Mapping - A visual type of outline, such as a flow chart
   d. Study Notes- Create small bits of information, index / flash cards work well

2. **Memory Techniques:**

   a. Study for short periods of time - (six 10 minute sessions are better than 1 hour)
   b. Divide bits of information into smaller odd-numbered lists - Split a list of 10 items into two smaller lists of 3 and 7
   c. Make associations - Imagine practical applications of information
   d. Create visual aids - Draw pictures, flow charts and arrows, etc.
   e. Say it out loud - Repeat aloud the information you are trying to memorize
   f. Use mnemonics - Most mnemonics or memory tricks are acronyms; words created from the first letter of each word in a series. (ex: ROY-G-BIV = Red, Orange. Yellow, Green, Blue, Indigo and Violet) make up your own!
   g. Create a "data dump" - Practice writing down material you have trouble recalling under pressure. Ask for a clean piece of paper once inside the exam room and "dump" this date before you even look at the first test question.
   h. Sleep with it and wake up with it! - Study immediately before you sleep (without interruption), and review immediately upon awakening

3. **Overcoming Test Anxiety**

   a. Reduce the general stress in your life
   b. Develop a well-organized daily /weekly routine
   c. Develop healthy lifestyle habits (exercise, diet, sleep, etc.)
   d. Affirm your ability (I am learning, I am knowledgeable, I am well-prepared)
   e. Confront your fears - by writing them down, with solutions
   f. Be overly prepared for your exam - it builds confidence!
   g. Do not allow yourself excuses for not following your plan or for procrastinating
   h. Visualize attaining your goals (licensure, personal & professional success, etc.)

4.   CONQUERING THE MULTIPLE CHOICE TEST

Multiple-choice tests are typically written to test either *cognition* (your thinking and reasoning ability) or *recognition* (your ability to remember or recognize material) with regard to a given subject area or topic. Professional test writers include the question "stem" or information on which the question is based and the various options or answer choices from which you must choose. Many test writers include "distracters," which can consist of extra language in the question (stem) portion, or very close options in the answer section. The more distractors used in test questions, the more the test will measure cognition. In other words, the distractor is used to prevent you from just "recognizing" the correct answer. Use of the following "answering strategies" can improve your multiple-choice test taking skills:

   a. Find the word, words or section of the stem which are "key" to understanding the real meaning of the question. What does the question really want to know? What are you really being asked? Eliminate any distracting portion of the question.

   b. Eliminate all clearly incorrect options. This means that you will now have to choose between fewer (but closer, more correct appearing) choices.

   c. Be aware of look-alike options. Some may actually be the opposite of the correct option, and yet appear to be correct at first glance.

   d. Guess if you must, but try first to eliminate the obviously incorrect options. Your "odds" are pretty good and leaving any question unanswered does you no service.

   e. Once you understand the question, go with your first impression. Do not change your answer unless you see that you have misunderstood the question.

   f. Answer the questions you are certain of first. You will have time to come back later to those questions which you are uncertain. You may actually find answers to those questions within other portions (or questions) of the exam.

   g. Check your test to make certain you have left no questions unanswered and that you answered each question the way you intended.

Remember, as in life ……….. you already know the answers,
the real test is to understand the questions.

CONTENT OUTLINE FOR STATE AND NATIONAL EXAMINATIONS

The NCBTMB and many other state licensure or certification examinations include questions from four major content areas. Examinations are "weighted" with regard to those areas of content. This means that a given percentage of questions within a test are taken from each content area. The following outlines represent the weighting of content areas by the NCBTMB as of June 1, 2005. The new NCETM test appears to cover the same material as the NCETMB test, omitting the material on Asian medicine and energy work. The following content area outlines are appropriate when reviewing material for any massage and bodywork licensure or certification examination. Please refer to the appropriate state certification agency for specific testing and licensure requirement details. A number of state and national certification/licensure body websites and phone numbers are provided for your convenience.

www.ncbtmb.com   (800) 296-0664

NCETMB Content Outline
160 questions, of which 150 will count toward the applicant's score

I. General Knowledge of Body Systems (16%)
A. Anatomy   B. Physiology   C. Pathology
1. Integumentary System
2. Skeletal System
3. Muscular System
4. Nervous System (including: Sympathetic & Parasympathetic Branches)
5. Endocrine System
6. Cardiovascular System
7. Lymphatic System & Immune Function
8. Urinary System, pH Balance, Fluid, & Electrolyte Balance
9. Respiratory System
10. Digestive System
11. Reproductive System
12. Craniosacral System
13. Energetic System
14. Meridian System

II. Detailed Knowledge of Anatomy, Physiology, and Kinesiology (26%)
A. Anatomy
1. Anatomical position and terminology
2. Individual muscles & groups
3. Muscle attachments
4. Muscle fiber direction
5. Tendons
6. Fascia
7. Joint structure
8. Ligaments
9. Bursae
10. Dermatomes
11. Primary and extraordinary meridians
12. Chakras

B. Physiology
    1. Response of the body to stress
    2. Basic nutritional principles
    3. Meridians / channels
C. Kinesiology & Biomechanics
    1. Actions of individual muscles & groups
    2. Types of muscle contractions
    3. Joint movements
    4. Movement patterns
    5. Proprioception

III. Clinical Pathology, including the recognition of signs & symptoms (12%)
A. Medical terminology
B. Etiology
C. Modes of contagious disease transmission
D. Signs & symptoms of disease
E. Psychological and emotional states
F. Effects of life stages
G. Effects of physical and emotional abuse & trauma
H. Factors that aggravate or alleviate disease
I. Physiological healing process
J. Indications and contraindications/cautions
K. Principles of acute versus chronic conditions
L. Stages / aspects of serious / terminal illness
M. Basic pharmacology
    1. Prescription medications
    2. Recreational drugs
    3. Herbs
    4. Natural supplements
N. Approaches used in Western medicine by other health professionals
O. Approaches used in Asian medicine by other health professionals

IV. Therapeutic Massage & Bodywork Assessment (18%)
A. Assessment methods
B. Assessing range of motion
C. Assessment areas
D. Somatic holding patterns
E. Posture analysis
F. Structural and functional integration
G. Ergonomic factors
H. Effects of Gravity (center of gravity, somatic patterns, balance/centering, etc.)
I. Proprioception of position & movement

V. Therapeutic Massage & Bodywork Application (22%)
A. Theory
    1. Effects / benefits of massage / bodywork
B. Methods and Techniques
    1. Client draping & positional support techniques
    2. Hydrotherapy / hydromassage application
    3. Stress management & relaxation techniques

4. Self-care activities for the client to maintain health
5. Principles of holistic practice / approach
6. Postural balancing
7. Use of massage and/or bodywork tools
8. Enhancing client's kinesthetic awareness
9. Joint movement techniques
10. Asian energy bodywork
11. Western energy bodywork
12. Static touch / holding
13. Techniques / strokes
14. Stretching
15. Aromatherapy
16. Topical analgesics
17. Gauging pressure as appropriate
18. Practitioner body mechanics
19. Standard precautions
20. CPR / first aid

VI. Professional Standards, Ethics, Business, and Legal Practices (6%)

A. Maintaining professional boundaries while responding to client's emotional needs
B. Client interviewing techniques
C. Communication with other health professionals
D. When to refer clients to other health professionals
E. Verbal and nonverbal communication skills
F. NCBTMB Code of Ethics & Standards of Practice
G. Issues of confidentiality
H. Legal & ethical parameters for scope of practice
I. Basic psychological & physical dynamics of practitioner / client relationship
J. Planning strategies for single & multiple sessions
K. Session record keeping practices
L. Basic business & accounting practices
M. Outsourcing business needs
N. Regulations pertaining to income reporting
O. Need for liability insurance
P. Stand & local credentialing requirements
Q. Legal entities

NCETM Content Outline
160 questions, of which 150 will count toward the applicant's score

I. General Knowledge of Body Systems (14%)
Refer to outline for NCETMB Section I, omitting the following:
12. Craniosacral System
13. Energetic System
14. Meridian System

II. Detailed Knowledge of Anatomy, Physiology, and Kinesiology (26%)
Refer to outline for NCETMB Section II, omitting the following:
A. 11. Primary and extraordinary meridians
12. Chakras
B. 3. Meridians / channels

III. Clinical Pathology, including the recognition of signs & symptoms (14%)
Refer to outline for NCETMB Section III, omitting the following:
O. Approaches used in Asian medicine by other health professionals

IV. Therapeutic Massage & Bodywork Assessment (16%)
Refer to outline for NCETMB Section IV

V. Therapeutic Massage & Bodywork Application (24%)
Refer to outline for NCETMB Section V, omitting the following:
B. 10. Asian energy bodywork
11. Western energy bodywork

VI. Professional Standards, Ethics, Business, and Legal Practices (6%)
Refer to outline for NCETMB Section VI

Ohio Massage Therapy Licensure Examination - www.med.ohio.gov/MT

A & P Section: 110 questions, of which 100 will count toward the applicant's score

SYSTEM	WHAT IS INCLUDED	APPROX. # OF QUESTIONS
Structure	Cells Tissues	3
Integument	Epidermis Dermis	5
Skeletal	Bone tissue-growth Axial Skeleton Appendicular skeleton Structure of bones	16
Joints	Of axial skeleton Of Appendicular skeleton Type of joint-motion	6
Muscular	Muscle tissue Reflexes and innervations Muscle contraction process Specific named muscles	35
Nervous	Spinal cord Brain & cranial nerves Sensory-motor integration Special senses Autonomic nervous system Peripheral (named) nerves Cellular structure	16
Endocrine	Generalized system Including targets Specific organs/hormones	4
Cardiovascular	Blood - Including Components, Heart, Vessels	10
Lymphatic	Specific organs Vessels, Cells and Immunology	5
Respiratory	Airways Lungs, including respiratory process Respiration, internal and external	5
Digestive	Mouth, esophagus, stomach Intestines Glands	3
Urinary	Kidneys Ureters, bladder, urethra	2
Total		**110**

Limited Branch Section: 110 questions, of which 100 will count toward the applicant's score

ISSUE TESTED	WHAT IS INCLUDED	APPROX. # OF QUESTIONS
Professionalism And Legal Issues	Professional Ethics – 4731-1-02 Scope of Practice – 4731-1-05 Legal Issues – 4731.22, 4731.34, 4731.41, 4731.99, Ohio Revised Code	5
Massage Techniques	Passive Touch/Pressure Touch Stroking/Effleurage Friction: Centripetal/Centrifugal Kneading/Petrissage Fulling Vibration Percussion Joint Movements	25
Effects of Massage	Mechanical/Direct Physical Effects Metabolic/Biochemical Effects Reflex/Neurological Effects Psychological Effects Effects by Technique	25
Therapeutic Applications for Massage	Conditions Disorders Diagnoses Applications of Various Techniques	30
Contraindications For Massage	Conditions Disorders Diagnoses Contraindication of Various Techniques Local and General Contraindications	10
Sanitation and Safety	Universal Precautions – Chapter 17, CDC (http://www.edc.gov/ncidod/hip/guide/overview.htm) Sanitation	5
Therapeutic Environment	Client Positioning/Draping and Comfort Lubricants	5
Hydrotherapy	Heat Applications Cold Applications Ice Therapy R.I.C.E. First Aid	5
Total		**110**

Texas Massage Therapy Registration Examination

Texas Department of Health (512) 834-6616

Content Area	Number of Questions
Swedish Massage Therapy (includes contraindications & pathology)	60
Anatomy and Physiology	60
Hydrotherapy	8
Business Practices and Professional Ethics	15
Health and Human Hygiene	7
Total	**150**

All questions in each content area are grouped together so you will not be constantly switching content areas during the exam. Each question has only one correct answer. Candidates will be required to answer multiple-choice questions, true/false questions and matching questions. The score will reflect the number of items that are answered correctly. There is no penalty for guessing. Candidates will have 2 ½ hours to complete the examination.

New York State Massage Therapy Licensure Examination

Content Area	Number of Questions	Percent
Assessment and Evaluation	20	14%
Development of a Treatment Plan	40	29%
Application of Treatment Skills	72	51%
Professional Responsibilities, Business Practice, & Professional Ethics	8	6%
Total	**140**	**100%**

The examination consists of 140 multiple-choice questions. Twenty (20) items test for knowledge of Eastern/Oriental teachings and methods. These items occur across the first three categories listed above.

The examination blueprint was prepared from practice analysis conducted in New York State in 2000 and became effective with the January 2002 examination. This is subject to change as practice analysis is updated.

Applicants for licensure in New York State will find information on the website of the Office of the Professions of the New York State Education Department: www.op.nysed.gov

For issues of practice: Massage Therapy Board Office: (518) 474-3817 ext. 150 or MSTHBD@mail.nysed.gov

For examination issues: Professional Examination Unit: (518) 474-3817 ext. 290 or OPEXAMS@mail.nysed.gov.

TABLE OF CONTENTS

See Section III-A, H - J for Massage Indications & Contraindications

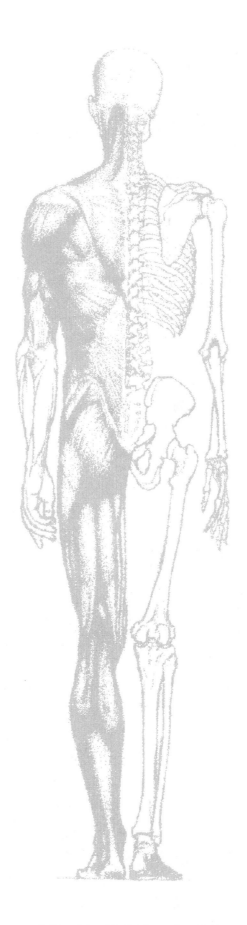

I-A   HUMAN ANATOMY, PHYSIOLOGY, AND KINESIOLOGY

A. Organization and Definitions:

Anatomical Position: The body is standing erect, face forward, arms at the sides, palms forward.

Anatomy: The science which studies the *structure* of an organism.

Anterior or Ventral: Toward the *front* of the body.

Cell: The simplest unit of living matter that can maintain life and reproduce itself.

Coronal or Frontal: A lengthwise plane running from side to side dividing the body or any of its parts into *anterior & posterior* sections

Distal: *Away* from or farthest from the trunk or the point of origin of a part.

Homeostasis: A *state of equilibrium* in which the internal environment of the body remains relatively constant.

Inferior or Caudal: Toward the *foot* end of the body - away from the head.

Kinesiology: The science which studies the *movement* of muscles.

Lateral: Toward the *side* of the body - away from the midline.

Medial: Toward the *midline* of the body.

Midsagittal: A lengthwise plane running from front to back dividing the body or any of its parts *equally* into *right and left halves*.

Organs: An organization of several different kinds of tissues so arranged that together they can perform a special function.

Physiology: The science which studies the *function* of an organism.

Posterior or Dorsal: Toward the *back* of the body (in humans).

Proximal: Toward or nearest the *trunk* of the body or the point of origin of a particular part.

Sagittal: A lengthwise plane running from front to back dividing the body or any of its parts into *right and left sides*.

Superior or Cranial: Toward the *head* end of the body.

Systems: An organization of varying numbers and kinds of *organs* so arranged that together they can perform complex functions for the body.

Tissues: An organization of a great many *similar cells* and varying amounts and kinds of non-living, intercellular substances between them.

Transverse: A crosswise plane dividing the body or any of its
(Horizontal) parts into *upper and lower sections*.

B. Cavities and the Organs That They Contain

    1. Dorsal Cavity - Contains the *cranial cavity*, which houses the *brain*, and the *spinal cavity*, which contains the *spinal cord*. This cavity is bounded by the cranial and spinal bones. (All cavities are bounded by *membranes*).

    2. Ventral Cavity - Consists of the *thoracic or chest cavity* and the *abdominopelvic cavity.*

        a. Thoracic or Chest Cavity - Contains a right and left pleural cavity & mid-portion called the *mediastinum*. A fibrous tissue wall around the mediastinum separates it from the right pleural sac, which houses the right lung, and the left pleural sac, which houses the left lung. The only organs not located in the mediastinum are the lungs. Organs located in the mediastinum are the: *heart, trachea, right & left bronchi, esophagus, thymus,* and *various blood vessels (i.e. thoracic aorta, superior vena cava), the thoracic duct and other lymphatic vessels, various lymph nodes, and nerves (i.e. phrenic & vagus).* The thoracic cavity is bounded by the sternum, ribs, spine, and *diaphragm*. The *diaphragm* separates the thoracic cavity and the abdominal cavity.

        b. Abdominopelvic Cavity - Comprises of an upper *abdominal* portion and a lower *pelvic* portion, extending from the diaphragm to the floor of the pelvis. The **abdominal cavity** contains the *liver, gallbladder, stomach, pancreas, intestines, spleen,* and *ureters.* The **pelvic cavity**, enclosed by the pelvic bones, contains the *bladder, certain reproductive organs (uterus, uterine tubes & ovaries in the female; prostate gland, seminal vesicles & par of vas deferens in the male), terminal end of the large intestine (sigmoid colon), and rectum.* **Note:** The *kidneys* are **not** located within a cavity. They are *retroperitoneal* – i.e.: located behind the peritoneum.

C. The Living Cell and its Parts:

    1. Cell - The smallest structure capable of maintaining life and reproducing. The outermost limit of the cell is the *plasma membrane*. This protein & lipid structure functions to maintain the wholeness of the cell and serves as a gateway through which chemicals may enter and leave. This membrane is *selectively permeable*, allowing some substances to pass while excluding others. The *cytoplasm* is the semi-fluid substance between the surface of the cell and its nucleus. Within the cytoplasm are membranes, which perform specific functions necessary for cell survival, known as *organelles*.

2. Cell Organelles & Their Functions

a. Endoplasmic Reticulum - Interconnected membranes with spaces between them forming canals; has openings to the outside of the cell and is connected to certain other organelles and to the nuclear membrane.

b. Ribosomes - Responsible for the synthesis of *protein molecules*.

c. Golgi Apparatus - Responsible for the synthesis of *carbohydrate molecules* for export from the cell.

d. Mitochondria - Energy source of the cell. *ATP synthesis*. "Powerhouse of the cell." Present in great numbers in muscle tissue.

e. Lysosomes - Capable of breaking down and digesting molecules of protein and carbohydrates when their enzymes are released. White blood cells have a great number of lysosomes.

f. Centrioles - Help form a spindle that appears during *mitosis* (cell division).

g. Cell Nucleus - Directs the activities of the cell; contains relatively large quantities of *DNA*.

3. External Organelles

a. Microvilli - *Tiny* hair-like projections of the cytoplasmic membrane located only in the *small intestine* to facilitate absorption by increasing surface area.

b. Cilia - *Small* hair-like projections of the cytoplasmic membrane located in the *respiratory system* acting to propel mucous upward.

c. Flagella - A single projection, such as found on a *sperm cell* allowing for propulsion of that cell.

4. Movements Through Cell Membranes

- The cell membrane functions as a gateway through which substances enter and leave the cell. Specifically, oxygen and food molecules enter a cell by passing through this membrane, while carbon dioxide and other wastes leave through it. This movement occurs both *passively* and *actively*.

a. Passive Transport Systems - A system in which movement occurs that does *not* require a direct expenditure of cellular energy.

1) Diffusion - Process by which molecules or ions scatter or spread themselves from regions of higher concentration to regions of lower concentration. They move continuously, rapidly, and in all directions. *Net Diffusion* is the movement of more particles of a substance in one direction than in the opposite direction. *Equal Diffusion* is the movement of the same number of solutes and water particles in each direction. *Equilibrium* is reached in both cases. During diffusion the cells are passive, not active and working. Cellular chemical reactions do not supply the energy that moves diffusing particles; the continual random movement of the molecules & ions supply this energy. (i.e. oxygen enters cells by diffusion through their membranes.) ***Facilitated Diffusion*** resembles both ordinary diffusion and active transport. Like ordinary diffusion, facilitated diffusion is a *carrier-mediated* process. In or near the outer surface of a cell membrane, a specific compound, the carrier, combines with the substance to be moved. The complex thus formed then rapidly diffuses through the membrane to its inner surface. There the carrier compound disassociates from the substance; it has fulfilled its function of facilitating (accelerating) the substance's diffusion through the membrane. This is one of the transports used in the small intestine.

2) Osmosis - The diffusion of *water (or any fluid)* through a selectively permeable membrane. Their concentration on both sides of the membrane eventually becomes equal.

3) Filtration - The physical process by which water & solutes pass through a membrane when a *hydrostatic pressure* is greater on one side of the membrane than the other. (*Hydrostatic pressure* is the force or weight of a fluid pushing against some surface.) Filtration always occurs *down* a hydrostatic pressure gradient and *only in one direction* through a membrane. Filtration is a major mechanism for moving substances through the membranous walls of blood capillaries; water and true solutes filter out of blood into the interstitial fluid in the microscopic spaces between the cells.

4) Dialysis - The diffusion of *solutes* through a selectively permeable membrane. It is the process where smaller molecules are separated from larger ones in a liquid. This process is employed in the "artificial kidney," by which the smaller molecules in the blood, such as urea, pass out through the cellophane membrane, while larger molecules, like those of blood proteins, remain inside.

b. Active Transport Systems - Requires the use of *ATP (energy)*. "Uphill" movement through a cell membrane, from an area of lower concentration to an area of higher concentration.

1) Permease System - *Cell (Ion) Pump*. Movement of molecules or ions against a concentration gradient. (i.e. Sodium-Potassium Pump.)

2) Pinocytosis - *Cell Drinking*. Process by which cells engulf tiny droplets of liquid from their surroundings.

3) Phagocytosis - *Cell Eating*. Process by which cells engulf solid particles, such as bacteria and cellular debris.

D. Tissues

Tissues are organizations of similar *cells* that specialize in one or more functions that serve the body as a whole. Composed of living cells separated by a non-living, intercellular substance (***matrix***). Although the cells of different tissues vary in size, shape, arrangement, and function, those within a tissue are similar in structure and function. There are four primary kinds of tissues:

1. Epithelial Tissue - Covers the body, organs, and surfaces, which are exposed to the outside as well as lining cavities. Serves as a protective barrier. Cells are packed closely together with very little intercellular material between them. *Avascular* - contains no blood vessels. Specializes in moving substances into and out of the blood (absorption & secretion). The cells undergo rapid division (*mitosis*), a fact of practical importance, so that old or destroyed epithelial cells can be replaced by new ones.

2. Connective Tissue - Most abundant & widely distributed in the body. Good structural material. Contains relatively few cells and a lot of *matrix*. Functions to *support* the body and its parts, to *connect* and hold them together, to *transport* substances through the body and to *protect* it from foreign invaders.

General Characteristics of Connective Tissue: Intercellular material predominates in most connective tissues and determines their physical characteristics; consists of fluid, gel, or solid matrix, with or without fibers (***collagenous, reticular, and elastic***). It connects *muscles to muscles, muscles to bones,* and *bones to bones*.

Main types of Connective Tissue

a. Reticular - Sheet-like (web-like) network of cells. Associated with the linings of blood vessels in the bone marrow, liver, spleen, and lymph nodes.

b. Areolar - (Glue) Widely distributed; composed of fibers in a loose, sticky gel and used to hold adjoining structures together.

c. Adipose - Consists of fat tissue to protect, insulate, and cushion internal organs.

d. Bone - Most rigid of the connective tissues due to the presence of mineral salts such as calcium phosphate and calcium carbonate; also contains a considerable amount of ***collagen.*** Hard and calcified.

e. Cartilage - "Gristle". Plastic-like material composed largely of fibers and a protein called *chondrin*. Functions to support parts, provide frameworks & attachments, and to protect underlying tissues.

f. Hemopoietic - Formation of blood & lymphatic cells in the red marrow cavities of bones. Important in the defense against disease.

g. Blood - *Vascular* tissue. Cells are suspended in a liquid intercellular matrix called *plasma*.

h. Dense Fibrous - Consists mainly of bundles of fibers arranged in parallel rows in a fluid/gel matrix. It contains relatively few *fibroblast cells*. This tissue is flexible but very strong. It composes ***tendons & ligaments***. Bundles of collagenous fibers endow tendons with great tensile strength and non-stretchability, desirable characteristics for these structures that anchor our *muscles to bones*. In ligaments, however, bundles of elastic fibers predominate. Hence, ligaments exhibit some degree of elasticity. Examples of dense fibrous connective tissue include: *tendons, ligaments, aponeurosis, deep fascia, scar, and capsule of kidney*.

3. Muscle Tissue - Specializes in movement and has the ability to contract. Moves the body and its parts. There are three types of muscle tissue: ***skeletal, cardiac,*** and ***visceral***. On the basis of nervous control, muscle is considered either *voluntary* or *involuntary*.

a. Skeletal Muscle is attached to bones. It is under *voluntary* control and its fibers are *striated* (alternating light & dark cross-markings producing visible lines or striae).

b. Cardiac Muscle composes the walls of the heart. It is *involuntary* and *striated*. At the end of the cell, where it touches another cell, is a band called an ***intercalated disc***, which only occurs in cardiac tissue.

     c. Visceral Muscle is in the walls of hollow internal structures such as blood vessels, intestines, uterus, stomach, urinary bladder, and many others. It is *involuntary* and *smooth*. It does not contain striations.

     4. Nervous Tissue - Specializes in rapid communication between various parts of the body and in integration of their activities. It is found in the *brain, spinal cord,* and *associated nerves*. The basic cells of this tissue are called **neurons,** which *transmit impulses* along cytoplasmic extensions to other neurons, muscles, or glands. In addition to neurons, nerve tissue contains **neuroglia,** which function to *support, insulate, bind,* and *protect* the neuron.

E. Membranes

Membranes constitute a special class of organs in that they are thin sheets of tissues covering or lining various parts of the body. Of the numerous membranes in the body, five kinds are discussed: ***mucous, serous, synovial, fascial,*** and ***cutaneous (skin)***.

     1. Mucous Membranes contain *epithelial cells* which line cavities or passageways of the body that *open to the exterior*, such as the lining of the mouth & entire digestive tract, the respiratory passages, and the genitourinary tracts. It consists, as do serous and cutaneous membranes, of a surface layer of epithelial tissue over a deeper layer of connective tissue. Mucous membranes perform the functions of *protection* (against microbial invasion), *secretion* (of mucous), and *absorption* of water, salts, and other solutes.

     2. Serous Membranes contain *epithelial cells* that line the *closed cavities of the body*, those that do not open to the exterior. The serous membrane which lines the thoracic cavity is called ***pleura***, that which lines the abdominal cavity is called ***peritoneum***, and that which lines the sac in which the heart lies is called ***pericardium***. It also covers the organs lying in these spaces. The term ***visceral layer*** is applied to the part of the membrane that covers the organs, whereas that which lines the cavity is called the ***parietal layer***. Between the two layers, there is a potential space kept moist by a small amount of *serous fluid*. When an organ moves against the body wall, (as the lungs do in respiration or when the heart beats in its serous sac), friction between the moving parts is reduced. The mechanical principle that moving parts must have lubricated surfaces is thereby carried out in the body.

     3. Synovial Membranes contain *connective tissue cells* that line ***joint capsules, tendon sheaths,*** and ***bursa***. Its smooth, moist surfaces also protect against friction.

     4. Fascial Membranes contain *connective tissue cells* and a semi-liquid, gel-like ground substance. Fascia covers, supports, and separates muscles and may be superficial, subcutaneous or deep.

5. Cutaneous (skin) Membranes contain *epithelial cells* and are composed of two main layers, the superficial and thinner layer known as the ***epidermis***, and the deeper and thicker layer known as the ***dermis***. The *epidermis* contains *melanocytes* which produce *melanin* (basic determinant of skin color), and *keratinocytes,* which produce *keratin* (fibrous waterproof protein). The *dermis* is composed largely of fibrous connective tissue, which includes tough white collagenous fibers & yellow elastin fibers. This gives the dermis its strength and elasticity. The dermis also contains the following structures:

    a. Hair - The part of the hair that is visible is the *shaft*, whereas that which is embedded in the dermis is the *root*. The root, together with its coverings (an outer connective tissue sheath & an inner epithelial coating that is a continuation of the stratum germinativum), forms the hair *follicle*. At the bottom of the follicle is a loop of capillaries enclosed in a connective tissue covering called the hair *papilla*.

    b. Nails - Produced by layers of specialized epithelial cells that are continuous with the epithelium of the skin. The keratin they contain is harder than that formed in the epidermis and hair follicles.

    c. Glands consist of epithelial cells specialized for synthesizing compounds which they secrete into either ducts or blood. *Endocrine glands* secrete into blood capillaries, and *exocrine glands* secrete into ducts that open on the surface of the epithelium.

    d. Sebaceous Glands secrete oil for the hair. Wherever hairs grow from the skin, there are at least two sebaceous glands for each hair. The oil or *sebum* secreted by these tiny glands has value not only because it keeps the hair supple, but it also keeps the skin soft & pliant. Moreover, it prevents excessive water evaporation from the skin and water absorption through the skin. Because fat is a poor conductor of heat, the sebum lessens the amount of heat lost from this large surface.

    e. Sweat Glands, although very small structures, are very important and very numerous, especially on the palms, soles, forehead, and axillae (armpits). Histologists estimate, for example, that a single square inch of skin on the palms of the hands contains about 3,000 sweat glands. Sweat secretion helps maintain homeostasis of fluid & electrolytes and body temperature. For example, if too much heat is being produced, as in strenuous exercise, or if the environmental temperature is high, these glands secrete more sweat, which in evaporating, cools the body surface. In as much as sweat contains some nitrogenous wastes, they also function as excretory organs. *Apocrine glands* are numerous in the armpits & groin, whereas *eccrine glands* are common on the forehead, neck, and back where they produce profuse sweating on hot days and during physical exercise.

f. Ceruminous Glands are thought to be modified sweat glands. They are located in the external ear canal. Instead of watery sweat, they secrete a waxy, pigmented substance called *cerumen*.

F. Organ Systems

1. The Skeletal System - Bones are the *organs* of the skeletal system. These organs, which are composed of several kinds of tissues, are classified according to their shapes and the ways they develop. Since they are rigid structures, bones provide support & protection for softer tissues, and they act together with skeletal muscles to make body movements possible. They also serve to manufacture blood cells & to store inorganic salts. The shapes of individual bones are closely related to their functions. Projections provide places for the attachments of muscles, tendons, and ligaments; openings serve as passageways for blood vessels, and nerves and the ends of bones, are modified to articulate with other bones at joints.

There are approximately 206 bones in the human skeleton, but the number may vary. The skeleton can be divided into two divisions: the **axial** portion which consists of the *skull, hyoid bone, vertebral column & thoracic cage*; and the **appendicular** portion which consists of the *pectoral girdle, arms, pelvic girdle & legs.*

a. Types of Bones & Examples of Each

1) Long Bones - Examples of long bones: bones of the upper and lower arm (humerus, ulna), of the thigh and leg (femur, tibia, and fibula), and of the fingers and toes (phalanges). A long bone consists of the following structures:

a) Diaphysis - The main shaft-like portion. Its hollow, cylindrical shape & thick compact bone, which composes it, adapts the diaphysis well to its function of providing strong support without cumbersome weight. Contains the *medullary cavity,* which is filled with marrow.

b) Epiphysis - Expanded portion at the end of each long bone, which articulates or forms a joint with another bone. Their shape is somewhat bulbous. This provides generous space for muscle attachments near joints & gives joints greater stability. Like a sponge, it is permeated by innumerable small spaces, hence its name *spongy* or *cancellous bone*. Because of the *porous* nature of this bone, and because the epiphyses have only a thin outer layer of dense, compact bone, they are lightweight structures for their size. *Marrow* fills the spaces of cancellous bone (yellow marrow in most adult epiphyses, but red marrow in the proximal epiphyses of the humerus & femur).

c) Articular Cartilage - The thin layer of *hyaline cartilage* that covers the articular or joint surfaces of the epiphysis. The resiliency of this material cushions jars and blows.

d) Periosteum - A tough covering of dense, white fibrous tissue that covers the bone except at joint surfaces, (where articular cartilage forms the covering). The periosteum is vascular and well innervated. Many of its fibers penetrate the underlying bone, welding these two structures to each other. (The penetrating fibers are called *Sharpey's fibers*.) Muscle tendon fibers interlace with periosteal fibers anchoring muscles firmly to bone. The periosteum contains many small blood vessels and numerous *osteoblasts* (bone-forming cells), in the inner layer of growing bones. Because its blood vessels send branches into the bone, the periosteum is essential for the nutrition of bone cells and therefore for their survival. Because of its osteoblasts, it is essential for both growth and repair of bones.

e) Medullary (marrow) Cavity - A tube-like hollow within the diaphysis of a long bone occupied by marrow. In the adult it contains mostly yellow marrow, which is a fat-storage tissue. In a child it contains mostly red marrow for the production of blood cells.

f) Endosteum - The membrane, which lines the medullary cavity of long bones. The endosteum contains clusters of *osteoblasts*. Until bone growth in length is complete, a layer of cartilage known as *epiphyseal cartilage* remains between each epiphysis and diaphysis. (**Note:** As *osteoblasts* are bone-forming cells by their action of placing calcium in bone, *osteoclasts* are cells which cause the erosion of bone by removing calcium from it.)

2) Short Bones - Wrist & ankle bones (carpals & tarsals).

3) Flat Bones - Certain bones of the cranium (frontals, occipital & parietals), sternum, ribs, scapula, and pelvis.

4) Irregular Bones - Bones of the spinal column (vertebrae, sacrum, coccyx), and certain bones of the skull (sphenoid, ethmoid & mandible).
Note: Some authorities recognize a fifth type of bone called *sesamoid* or *round* bones. They are usually small & occur within tendons adjacent to joints. (patella; distal end, inferior surface of 1st metatarsal).

b. Bony Landmarks

1) Projections of bone - sites for muscle attachment

a) Tuberosity - Large, rounded projection may be roughened.

b) Tubercle - Small, rounded knob-like process (supraglenoid tubercle of the scapula).

c) Trochanter - Very large, blunt, irregular process only on femur.

d) Crest - Narrow ridge of bone, usually prominent (iliac crest of ilium).

e) Line - Narrow ridge of bone, less prominent than a crest (linea aspera of the posterior femur).

f) Epicondyle - Raised area on or above a condyle.

g) Spine - Sharp, slender, often pointed projection.

h) Malleolus -Medial & lateral projections at the distal ends of the tibia & fibula (i.e. anklebones).

i) Process - A prominent projection on a bone (i.e. mastoid process of the temporal bone).

2) Projections of bone that help to form joints

a) Head - Bony expansion carried on a narrow neck; an enlargement on the end of a bone that usually articulates with another bone (i.e. head of the humerus).

b) Facet - Smooth, nearly flat articular surface (i.e. costal facet of a thoracic vertebra).

c) Condyle - Rounded process that usually articulates with another bone (i.e. occipital condyle).

d) Ramus - Arm-like bar of bone (i.e. ramus of the mandible).

e) Suture - A line of union between bones (i.e. lambdoidal suture between the occipital & parietal bones).

3) Depressions & openings in bone allowing blood vessels & nerves to pass

a) Meatus - A tube like passageway within a bone (i.e. auditory meatus).

b) Sinus - Cavity within a bone, filled with air and lined with mucous membrane.

c) Fossa - Shallow, basin-like depression in a bone, often serving as an articular surface.

d) Groove - Furrow in bone (i.e. bicipital groove).

e) Fissure - Narrow, slit-like opening.

f) Foramen - Round or oval opening through a bone that usually serves as a passageway for blood vessels, nerves, or ligaments (i.e. foramen magnum of the occipital bone).

c. Five Functions of Bones

1) Support - Bones serve as the supporting framework of the body much as steel girders function as the supporting framework of buildings.

2) Protection - Hard, bony "boxes" protect delicate structures enclosed by them. (i.e. the skull protects the brain, and the rib cage protects the lungs & heart.)

3) Movement - Bones with their joints constitute levers. Muscles are anchored firmly to bones. As muscles contract & shorten, force is applied to the bony levers and movement results.

4) Reservoir (Storage) - Bones serve as the major reservoir into which calcium is deposited, or from which it is withdrawn as needed to maintain the homeostasis of blood calcium, a vitally important condition.

5) Hemopoiesis - The process of blood cell formation. Tissues that carry on this process are specialized connective tissues of two kinds, *myeloid tissue* and *lymphatic tissue*. (Red bone marrow is another name for myeloid tissue.) In the adult, it is only found in a few bones in the sternum and ribs, in the bodies of the vertebrae, in the diploe of the cranial bones, and in the proximal epiphyses of the femur and humerus. Red marrow occurs in many more bones in newborn infants and children. Because it forms blood cells, red bone marrow is one of the most important tissues of the body. Its very location, hidden in the bones like valuables in a safety deposit box, suggests its vital importance.

d. Skeletal System Articulations

Articulations or **joints** are junctions between bones. They are classified according to the amount of movement they make possible.

1) Synarthroses - Occur between bones that come into close contact with one another. A thin layer of *fibrous* tissue separates the bones at these joints. No active *(very slight)* movement takes place. (i.e. the *suture* between a pair of flat bones of the cranium.)

2) Amphiarthroses - Slightly movable joints. They are connected by discs of *cartilage*. (i.e. between the ribs & sternum, the vertebrae in the vertebral column, and the symphysis pubis.)

3) Diarthroses - Freely movable joints. The ends of bones are held together by a joint capsule composed of an outer layer of ligaments and an inner layer of synovial membrane, which secrets synovial fluid to act as a joint lubricant. For this reason, freely movable joints are also called *synovial* joints. This is our most numerous type of joint.

Characteristics of diarthrotic joints include:

a) Joint Capsule - Sleeve-like extension of the periosteum of each of the articulating bones. The capsule completely encases the ends of the bones and binds them to each other.

b) Synovial Membrane - Moist, slippery membrane that lines the inner surface of the joint capsule. It attaches to the margins of the articular cartilage and secretes *synovial fluid*, which lubricates the inner joint surfaces.

c) Articular Cartilage - *Hyaline cartilage* that covers and cushions the articulating ends of the bones.

d) Joint Cavity - Small space between the articulating surfaces of the two bones of a joint. Because of this cavity with no tissue growing between the articulating surfaces of the bones, the bones are free to move against one another.

e) Ligaments - Strong cords of dense, white, fibrous tissue at most synovial joints. These grow between the bones, lashing them even more firmly together than possible with the joint capsule alone.

Examples of diarthrotic joints include:

a) Ball & Socket Joints (multiaxial) - Those in which a ball-shaped head of one bone fits into a concave socket of another bone (i.e. the shoulder and hip joints). Of all the joints in our bodies, the ball & socket joints permit the widest range of movements, namely *flexion, extension, abduction, adduction, rotation,* and *circumduction*.

b) Ellipsoidal Joints (multiaxial) - Those in which an oval-shaped condyle fits into an elliptical socket. The radius joins the carpal bones (scaphoidlunate and triquetrum) by means of an ellipsoidal joint, which permits the movements of *flexion & extension* of the hand in one axis, and movement of a*bduction* and *adduction* in another axis. This is known as *biaxial* movement. **Note:** Next to the ball & socket joints, ellipsoidal joints allow the widest range of movements. (also known as condyloid joints)

c) Saddle Joints (biaxial) - Like ellipsoidal joints, permit biaxial movements. The shapes of the articulating ends of the bones, however, differ in the two types of joints. In the saddle joint, a saddle-shaped surface of one bone fits into a saddle-shaped surface of another bone. Only *one* pair of saddle joints exists in the body, one in each hand *between the metacarpal and carpal bones of the thumb* called the *trapezium*. These are deservedly famous joints, at least to anatomists. They make possible the great mobility of the human thumbs. We can ***flex, extend, abduct, and adduct*** them. But most importantly of all, we can ***oppose*** them (i.e. move out thumbs to touch the tip of any one of our fingers). If we did not have a saddle joint at the base of each thumb, we could not oppose the thumb and would be unable to do such simple things as picking up a pin or grasping a pencil between the thumb and forefinger.

d) Hinge Joints (uniaxial) - Permit only *flexion* and *extension* movements, which might be called hinged-door movements (i.e. bending the elbow).

e) Pivot Joints (uniaxial) - Those in which a small projection of one bone pivots in an arch of another bone, causing the first bone to ***rotate*** on its axis. There are two pivot joints in the body, one between the first two cervical vertebrae (atlas & axis), and the other between the proximal ends of the radius & ulna.

f) Gliding Joints (uniaxial) - Allow only the simplest type of motion, specifically, a little ***gliding*** back and forth or sideways. These include most of the joints between both the carpal and tarsal bones, and also all of the joints between the articular processes of the vertebrae (includes: *facet* type joints).

e. Definitions of Movement

1) Flexion - *Decreases* the size of the angle between the anterior surfaces of articulating bones. (Exception: flexion of the knee and the joints decrease the angle between the posterior surfaces of the articulated bones.) Flexing movements are *bending* or *folding* movements (i.e. bending the head forward is flexion of the joint between the occipital bone and the atlas; bending the elbow is flexion of the elbow joint or of the lower arm). Flexing movements of the arms and legs may be thought of as "withdrawing" movements.

2) Lateral Flexion - *Decreasing* the size of the angle between the lateral surfaces of the body (i.e. lateral flexion of the trunk brings the trunk closer to the hip).

3) Extension - The return from flexion. *Increases* the size of the angle between articulating bones. Extension restores a part to its *anatomical position* from the flexed position. Examples of extension would include: returning the head to its upright anatomical position from its flexed, bent forward position; unbending the elbow thus returning the forearm to its anatomical position. Continuation of extension beyond anatomical position is called *hyperextension*. Hyperextension of the head would be stretching it backward from the upright position; of the arm, bringing the humerus straight back behind the body.

4) Abduction - Moves a bone *away* from the midline of the body (i.e. moving the arms straight out to the sides).

5) Adduction - Moves a bone *toward* the midline of the body (i.e. bringing the arms back to the sides).

6) Horizontal Adduction - Moves a bone *toward* the midline of the body at a horizontal level (i.e. raising the humerus and bringing it across the chest).

7) Rotation - The pivoting of a bone on its own axis somewhat as a top turns on its axis (i.e. holding the head in an upright position and turning it from one side to the other).

8) Inversion - Turns the sole of the foot inward (see below as supination).

9) Eversion - Turns the sole of the foot outward (see below as pronation).

10) Circumduction - Causes the bone to describe the surface of a cone as it moves. The distal end of the bone describes a circle. It combines flexion, abduction, extension, and adduction in succession (i.e. describing a circle with the arms outstretched).

11) Supination - Movement of the forearm that turns the palm forward, as it is in anatomical position (adduction + inversion = supination of the foot).

12) Pronation - Turning the forearm so as to bring the back of the hand forward, palms down (abduction + eversion = pronation of the foot).

13) Elevation - Raising a part (i.e. shrugging the shoulders).

14) Depression - Lowering a part (i.e. drooping the shoulders).

15) Protraction - Moving a part forward (i.e. thrusting the chin forward).

16) Retraction - Moving a part backward (i.e. pulling the chin backward).

* See Range of Motion Chart on Page 58

2. The Muscular System

Muscles, the *organs* of the muscular system, account for nearly half of the body weight. They consist largely of muscle cells, which have become differentiated into contractile units and can be stimulated by the actions of certain nerve cells to contract. As was mentioned previously, there are three types of muscle tissue: *skeletal, cardiac,* and *visceral*.

a. Anatomy of Skeletal Muscle

1) Skeletal Muscle is usually fastened to bones. Its fibers are *striated* and under *voluntary* control.

2) Composed of nerve, vascular, and various connective tissues as well as striated muscle tissue. Each fiber represents a single muscle cell, which is the unit of contraction. Muscle fibers are cylindrical cells with numerous nuclei and are grouped into bundles by **fascia**. The protein **myofilaments** (*actin & myosin*) within a muscle cell contract towards each other causing movement. *Calcium* and *ATP* are necessary for this action. Striations, cross-bands, are produced by the arrangement of the actin & myosin filaments.

3) Muscle fibers are stimulated to contract by *motor neurons*. The area of contact between a muscle fiber and nerve is known as the *motor end-plate* or *neuro-muscular junction*. ATP supplies the energy for muscle fiber contraction. Muscle cells contain a great many mitochondria.

b. Three General Functions of Skeletal Muscle

1) Movement - Skeletal muscle contractions produce movement either of the body as a whole or of its parts (i.e. walking, talking, breathing, swallowing, facial expressions).

2) Heat Production - Muscle cells, like all cells, produce heat by the process known as *catabolism* (the break down of larger molecules into smaller ones). Because skeletal muscle cells are both highly active and numerous, they produce a major share of total body heat. Skeletal muscle contractions, therefore, constitute one of the most important parts of the mechanism for maintaining homeostasis of temperature.

3) Posture - The continued partial contraction of many skeletal muscles makes possible standing, sitting, and other maintained positions of the body.

c. Types of Muscular Contractions

1) Tonic (Tone) - A continual, partial contraction. At any one moment a small number of the total fibers in a muscle contract, producing tautness of the muscle rather than a recognizable contraction and movement.

2) Isotonic - (iso = same; tonic = tone, pressure, or tension) A contraction in which the tone or tension within a muscle remains the same, but the length of the muscle changes, producing movement and doing work. *Concentric*: muscle contraction in which the muscle fibers shorten (i.e. flexion of elbow in lifting a weight) and *eccentric*: muscle contraction in which the muscle fibers lengthen with resistance (resistance of flexors in extension of elbow when lowering a weight).

3) Isometric - (iso = same; metric = measurement) A contraction in which muscle length remains the same, but in which muscle tension increases. The muscle will tighten, but will not produce movement or do work (i.e. pushing your arm against a wall and feeling the tension increase in your arm muscle).

4) Fibrillation - An abnormal type of contraction in which individual fibers contract asynchronously, producing a flutter of the muscle but no effective movement (i.e. fibrillation of the heart occurs fairly often).

5) Twitch - A single quick, jerky muscular contraction from a single nerve impulse followed by relaxation.

6) Tetanic - A continuous, forceful muscular contraction arising from a series of at least 30 nerve impulses per second. (also known as a spasm or cramp)

d. Definitions of Importance

1) Threshold Stimulus - Minimal stimulus needed to elicit a muscular contraction.

2) All-or-None Response - If a muscle fiber (cell) contracts at all, it will contract completely (all the way).

3) Prime Mover - The muscle or muscles whose contraction is mainly responsible for a particular body movement.

4) Antagonist - The muscle or muscles that relax while the prime mover is contracting to produce the movement. (exception: contraction of the antagonist at the same time as the prime mover when some part of the body needs to be held rigid, such as the knee joint when standing.)

5) Synergist - Muscle or muscles that contract at the same time as the prime mover. They may help the prime mover produce its movement or stabilize a part, hold it steady, so that the prime mover produces a more effective movement.

6) Fixator (Stabilizer) - The muscle or muscles responsible for stabilizing the non-moveable part of a joint so other muscles can contract to produce a certain movement (i.e. the shoulder joint being held immobile while the biceps are contracting to flex the forearm).

7) Neutralizer - Counteracts the action of another muscle to prevent undesirable movements.

8) Tendon - A strong, tough cord of white fibrous connective tissue that connects a muscle to a bone. It is continuous with the fibrous covering of bone, (periosteum) and fascia of muscle. The fibrous wrapping of a muscle may extend as a broad, flat sheet of connective tissue known as an *aponeurosis*, to attach it to adjacent structures, usually the fibrous wrappings of another muscle.

9) Bursae - Small connective tissue sacs lined with synovial membrane and containing synovial fluid. Bursae are located wherever pressure is exerted over moving parts (i.e. between skin and bone, between tendons and bone, between muscles and bones, or ligaments and bone). They act as cushions, relieving pressure between moving parts. Some bursae that fairly frequently become inflamed (*bursitis*) are as follows: *subacromial bursa*, between the head of the humerus and the acromion process and the deltoid muscle; *olecranon bursa*, between the olecranon process of the ulna and the skin; *prepatellar bursa*, between the patella and the skin. Inflammation of the pre-patellar bursa is known as housemaid's knee, whereas olecranon bursitis is called student's elbow.

e. Scapulo-humeral Muscles

Muscle	Origin	Insertion	Action
Trapezius	Occipital Bone C7 - T12 (spinous processes) *(Most superficial back muscle)*	Clavicle Scapula	Elevation, upward rotation & retraction of scapula. Extends head when occipital acts as insertion.
Serratus Anterior	Outer surface of upper 8 ribs	Scapula	Pulls shoulder forward; protracts & rotates it upward. Stabilizes scapula against chest wall. *(Weakness is evidenced by "winged" scapula.)*
Pectoralis Major	Clavicle, Sternum Costal Cartilage of upper 6 ribs	Humerus (bicipital groove)	Flexes upper arm; adducts upper arm anteriorly; draws it across chest. *(Horizontal adduction.)* Medial rotation of humerus.
Pectoralis Minor	Anterior 3,4,5, ribs	Scapula (coracoid)	Pulls shoulder down and forward. Abducts scapula. *(Lies in close proximity & superficial to brachial plexus & subclavian artery, hypertonicity: may present with rounded shoulders & elicit symptoms of numbness, weakness or pain in associated upper extremity)*
Latissimus Dorsi	Aponeurosis from T7 to Iliac Crest, Lower 3 or 4 ribs, Inferior angle of Scapula.	Humerus (bicipital groove)	Extends upper arm; adducts upper arm posteriorly; medial rotation of arm.
Teres Major	Scapula	Humerus (bicipital groove)	Assists Latissumus Dorsi in extension, adduction and medial rotation of arm.
Deltoid	Clavicle, Scapula	Humerus (deltoid tuberosity)	Abducts upper arm; assists flexion & medial rotation of humerus.

e. Scapulo-humeral Muscles: (continued)

Muscle	Origin	Insertion	Action
Levator Scapula	C1 - C4 (transverse processes)	Scapula	Elevation & downward rotation of scapula.
Rhomboids	C7 - T5 (spinous processes)	Scapula	Retraction & downward rotation of scapula.
Supraspinatus	Scapula	Humerus	Stabilizes head of humerus & initiates abduction of humerus.
Infraspinatus	Scapula	Humerus	Rotates arm outward *(lateral rotation)*; extension of humerus.
Teres Minor	Scapula	Humerus	Rotates arm outward; extension of humerus.
Subscapularis	Scapula	Humerus	Rotates arm medially. (works with anterior deltoid & pectoralis major in this action.)
			(Supraspinatus, Infraspinatus, Teres Minor and Subscapularis compromise the SITS muscle group, or Rotator Cuff.)
Biceps Brachii	Scapula	Radius	Flexion of humerus. Supination of hand.
Brachialis	Humerus	Ulna	Flexes forearm at the elbow. (Strongest elbow flexor.)
Coracobrachialis	Scapula	Humerus	Flexion; adduction of humerus.
Brachioradialis	Humerus	Radius	Flexion of elbow.
Triceps Brachii	Scapula, Humerus	Ulna	Extends lower arm. (ulna) Extension of humerus.

f. Muscles that move the Hip, Thigh, Lower Leg, and Foot

Muscle	Origin	Insertion	Action
Iliopsoas	Iliac Fossa, Lumar Vertebrae *(rotates hip at SI joint)*	Femur (lessor trochanter)	Flexion of hip. Assists in abduction & lateral rotation of thigh.
Gluteus Maximus	Ilium, Sacrum, Coccyx	Femur (greater trochanter & ITB)	Forceful extension of hip. Lateral rotation of extended hip.
Gluteus Medius	Ilium	Femur	Abducts and rotates thigh medially.
Gluteus Minimus	Ilium	Femur	Abducts & rotates thigh medially; stabilizes pelvis on femur.
Tensor Fasciae Latae	Ilium	Tibia (via ITB) *(may be involved with Gluteus Max. in ITB Syndrome)*	Assists abduction of thigh & braces knee in walking.
Quadratus Lumborum	Iliac Crest *(commonly involved in low back pain)*	Lumbar Vertebrae	Raises hip *or* lateral flexion of trunk.
Piriformis	Anterior Sacrum *(Lies in close proximity, superficial to the sciatic nerve)*	Femur	Rotates thigh outward. Abducts & extends thigh.
Adductor Brevis	Pubic Bone	Femur	Adducts thigh.
Adductor Longus	Pubic Bone	Femur	Adducts thigh.
Adductor Magnus	Pubic Bone	Femur	Adducts thigh.
Gracilis	Pubic Bone	Tibia	Adducts thigh; assists flexion & medial rotation of flexed knee.
Sartorius	Ilium *(This is longest muscle in body)*	Tibia	Weakly flexes thigh & leg, adducts leg. Rotates thigh laterally & leg medially. Assists in crossing of the leg.

f. Muscles that move the Hip, Thigh, Lower Leg and Foot (continued)

Muscle	Origin	Insertion	Action
Rectus Femoris	Ilium, Acetabulum of Femur *(Most superficial quadriceps muscle)*	Tibia	Flexes thigh; extends leg at knee.
Vastus Lateralis	Femur	Tibia	Extends leg at knee.
Vastus Medialis	Femur	Tibia	Extends leg at knee.
Vastus Intermedius	Femur	Tibia	Extends leg at knee.
Biceps Femoris	Ischial Tuberosity, Femur *(Most superficial hamstring muscle)*	Fibula	Flexes & rotates leg laterally and extends thigh.
Semitendinosus	Ischial Tuberosity	Tibia	Flexes & rotates leg medially and extends thigh.
Semimembranosus	Ischial Tuberosity *(Most medial hamstring muscle)*	Tibia	Flexes & rotates leg medially and extends thigh.
Gastrocnemius	Femur	Calcaneus	Extends foot *(plantar flexion)*, *or* flexes lower leg, not both simultaneously.
Soleus	Tibia, Fibula	Calcaneus	Extends foot (strongest *plantar flexor* of ankle).
Tibialis Anterior	Tibia	Tarsal and Metatarsal	*Dorsiflexion* of ankle; inversion of foot. Contributes to forming the "arch" of foot.
Tibialis Posterior	Tibia, Fibula	Tarsal and Metatarsal	*Plantar flexion* of ankle; inversion of foot. Contributes to forming the "arch" of foot.
	(Tibialis Ant. & Post. commonly involved in "shin splints")		
Popliteus	Femur	Tibia	Initiates "unlocking" of extended knee by medial rotation of tibia.

g. Muscles of the Abdominal Wall

Muscle	Origin	Insertion	Action
Rectus Abdominis	Costal cartilage of ribs 5,6,7,; Xiphoid Process	Pubis	Flexes trunk; compresses abdominal contents.
External Oblique	Lower 8 ribs	Iliac Crest Linea Alba	Flexion of trunk to opposite side; compresses abdominal contents.
Internal Oblique	Iliac Crest Inguinal Ligament	Lower 4 ribs Linea Alba	Flexion of trunk to same side; compresses abdominal contents.
Transverse Abdominis	Lower ribs; Iliac Crest; Fascia	Pubic Bone Linea Alba	Compresses abdominal contents.

h. Muscles that move the Head

Muscle	Origin	Insertion	Action
Sternocleido-mastoid	Sternum Clavicle	Temporal Bone	*Bilaterally* - flexes head. *Unilaterally* - lateral flexion or rotation of head to opposite side.
Scalenes	Cervical Vertebrae	1st & 2nd rib	*Bilaterally* - flexes head. *Unilaterally* - lateral flexion of head to same side. Can also raise ribs in inspiration.
	(The brachial plexus and subclavian artery pass between the anterior & middle scalenes.)		
Splenius Capitis Splenius Cervicis	C7 - T6 (spinous processes)	Temporal & Occipital Bones; C1-3	*Bilaterally* - Extension of head. *Unilaterally* - rotation of head to same side.
Erector Spinae	Vertebral Column	Occipital & Temporal Bones	Extension of spine; lateral flexion of spine.

i. Muscles of Mastication (Chewing)

Muscle	Origin	Insertion	Action
Masseter	Zygomatic Arch	Mandible	Raises (closes) jaw; assists protraction of jaw.
Pterygoid *(internal/medial)*	Sphenoid, Palatal	Mandible & Maxilla	Raises jaw; pulls jaw sideways.
Temporalis	Temporal Bone	Mandible	Raises and retracts jaw.
Buccinator	Maxilla & Mandible	Lips	Maintains cheeks near teeth

j. Diaphragm - This muscle of importance *separates thoracic and abdominal cavities*. It contracts vertically downward in inspiration and relaxes in expiration. There are three openings to allow for passage of the **esophagus, inferior vena cava,** and **aorta**.

3. The Nervous System:

The actions of all body parts; cells, tissues, organs, and systems, must be directed toward a single goal in order to survive, the maintenance of *homeostasis*. The general task of controlling & coordinating body activities is handled by the nervous and endocrine systems. The nervous system provides *rapid* and *precise* control of muscles and glands.

a. Anatomy of the Nervous System

The nervous system consists of the **brain, spinal cord,** and numerous **peripheral nerves.** Nervous tissue consists of masses of nerve cells called *neurons.* These are highly specialized cells that are capable of transmitting nerve impulses to other neurons or to cells outside of the nervous system. Between these cells and fibers are *neuroglial cells* which function much like connective tissue in that they support, bind, and protect the neuron.

The **neuron** consists of a *cell body, dendrites,* and one *axon*. Dendrites, with their many branches, conduct nerve impulses toward the cell body. The distal ends of dendrites of *sensory neurons* are called *receptors* because they receive the stimuli that initiates conduction. The *axon* is a single process that extends out from the neuron cell body and carries impulses away from the cell body. The **myelin sheath**, a segmented wrapping around a nerve fiber, consists of *myelin*, a fatty substance. This is only found on *motor neurons* and increases the rate of an *impulse*. A **synapse** is the microscopic space between the axon of one neuron and the dendrite of another.

b. Three Basic Types of Neurons & Their Functions

1) Sensory (afferent) Neurons - Transmit nerve impulses *to* the spinal cord or brain from peripheral body parts.

2) Motor (efferent) Neurons - Transmit nerve impulses ***away*** from the brain or spinal cord to muscle or glandular tissues.

3) Interneurons - Conduct impulses from sensory to motor neurons. Interneurons lie *entirely* within the central nervous system (brain & spinal cord).

The nervous system consists of billions of cells and is astoundingly complex. The *organs* include the brain, spinal cord, and various nerves. These parts are divided into a ***Central Nervous System***, which consists of the *brain and spinal cord*, and a ***Peripheral Nervous System***, which consists of the nerves that connect the brain and spinal cord to all body parts.

c. The Central Nervous System

The **Central Nervous System** consists of the ***brain and spinal cord***. The brain lies within the *cranial cavity* of the skull, and the spinal cord, which is continuous with the brain, occupies the *vertebral canal* within the vertebral column. Beneath these bony coverings, the brain and spinal cord are protected by membranes called ***meninges*** that are located between the bone and the soft tissues of the nervous system. The **meninges** have three layers: the ***dura mater***, the ***arachnoid,*** and the ***pia mater***.

Dura Mater - The outermost layer composed primarily of tough, white fibrous connective tissue. It lines the cranial cavity and forms an internal periosteum where it attaches to the surrounding skull bones. The dura mater continues into the vertebral canal as a strong sheath that surrounds the spinal cord.

Arachnoid - A thin, netlike membrane located between the dura mater and pia mater. It spreads over the brain and spinal cord. Between the arachnoid mater and pia mater is a watery fluid known as ***cerebrospinal fluid***.

Pia Mater - The innermost layer consisting of blood vessels, which aid in nourishing the underlying cells of the brain and spinal cord.

The anatomical structures of the Central Nervous System include:

1) Brain - The largest and most complex part of the nervous system. It occupies the cranial cavity and is composed of billions of neurons and innumerable nerve fibers. The neurons communicate with one another and with neurons in other parts of the system. The brain can be divided into four major portions: *cerebrum, cerebellum, diencephalon,* and the *brain stem*:

a) Cerebrum - The largest and uppermost division of the brain. Consists of two large lobes, the right and left *cerebral hemispheres*, which are mirror images of each other. The lobes of the cerebral hemispheres are named after the skull bones that they underlie. They include the *frontal lobe,* which forms the anterior portion of each and lies below and lateral to the frontal lobe, and the *occipital lobe,* which forms the posterior portion of each cerebral hemisphere. The surface of the cerebrum is made up of gray matter, composed of millions of axon terminals synapsing with millions of dendrites and cell bodies of other neurons. The large interior of the cerebrum consists mostly of white matter made up of numerous tracts, with areas of gray matter lying deep inside.

b) Cerebellum - The second largest part of the brain, located just below the posterior portion of the cerebrum. The cerebellum consists of two large lateral masses, the *cerebellar hemispheres*, and a central section. As in the cerebrum, gray matter makes up the outer portion and white matter predominates in the interior.

c) Diencephalon - Located between the cerebrum and the midbrain and generally surrounds the third ventricle. It is composed largely of gray matter organized into nuclei. It consists of several structures, the main ones being the *thalamus* and *hypothalamus*.

d) Brain Stem - A bundle of nerve tissue that extends downward from the base of the *cerebrum* to the level of the *foramen magnum*. It is the first part of the brain to develop from the spinal cord. It is composed of numerous tracts of myelinated nerve fibers and several masses of gray matter (*nuclei*). This structure is composed of three divisions: *medulla, pons, and midbrain*.

(1) Medulla - Part formed by the enlargement of the spinal cord as it enters the cranial cavity through the foramen magnum. Consists of white matter, (*ascending and descending tracts*), and a mixture of gray and white matter, (*reticular formation*). Extends from the level of the foramen magnum to the pons. Because of its location, all ascending and descending nerve fibers must pass through the medulla. (Note: The *medulla* is also known as *medulla oblongata*.)

(2) Pons - Lies just above the medulla, separating the medulla from the midbrain. Composed of *ascending and descending tracts* making up the white matter of pons; contains a small amount of gray matter (*nuclei*).

(3) Midbrain - Lies just above the pons, below the diencephalon and cerebrum. Contains ascending and descending tracts and a few nuclei. The bundles of myelinated nerve fibers (*cerebral peduncles*) join lower parts of the brain stem and spinal cord to the cerebrum. *Corpora quadrigemin*, two superior and two inferior *colliculi*, are rounded eminences on the dorsal surface of the midbrain. Red nucleus lies in the gray matter of the midbrain. *Cerebral aqueduct* is the fluid-filled space located in the midbrain.

2) Spinal Cord: A slender nerve column within the spinal cavity continuous with the brain. The spinal cord is said to begin where the nerve tissue leaves the cranial cavity at the level of the foramen magnum, and terminates near the intervertebral disk that separates the first and second lumbar vertebrae, where it tapers off to a point. (The spinal cord does not completely fill the spinal cavity. It also contains the meninges, spinal fluid, a cushion of adipose tissue, and blood vessels.) Composed of *thirty-one* segments, each giving rise to a pair of *spinal nerves,* which branch out to various body parts and connect them with the central nervous system. The neck region contains a bulge called the *cervical enlargement*, which gives off nerves to the arms. A similar thickening in the lower back, the *lumbar enlargement*, gives off nerves to the legs. The spinal cord consists of a core of gray matter surrounded by white matter. The *central canal* is continuous with the ventricles of the brain and contains *cerebrospinal fluid*.

The physiology of the Central Nervous System:

1) Cerebrum - Concerned with the higher brain functions. It contains centers for interpreting sensory impulses arriving from various sense organs as well as centers for initiating voluntary muscular movements. It stores the information of memory and can utilize this information for the process of reasoning. It is the area for conscious thought, emotions, language functions, and in determining a person's intelligence and personality.

2) Cerebellum - Performs three general functions, all of which have to do with the control of skeletal muscles. It acts to produce skilled movements by coordinating the activities of groups of muscles, controls skeletal muscles so as to maintain equilibrium, and helps to control posture. It functions below the level of consciousness to make movements smooth and steady instead of jerky and uncoordinated.

3) Diencephalon - Produces conscious recognition of the crude, less critical sensations of pain, temperature and touch. Plays a part in emotions by associating sensory impulses with feelings of pleasantness and unpleasantness, arousal or alerting, and complex reflex movements. Serves as a regulator and coordinator of autonomic activities associated with water balance, sleep, appetite, body temperature, and sexual arousal.

4) Brain Stem - Performs sensory, motor, and reflex functions. Concerned with regulating *vital functions* such as the cardiac, respiratory, and vasomotor centers. Also contains reflex centers for eye movements, coughing, sneezing, hiccupping, swallowing, and vomiting.

5) The Spinal Cord - Performs two general functions, to conduct nerve impulses and to serve as a center for spinal reflexes. The *tracts* of the spinal cord provide a two-way system of communication between the brain and parts outside the nervous system. *Ascending tracts* conduct impulses from body parts and carry sensory information to the brain. *Descending tracts* conduct motor impulses from the brain to muscles and glands.

d. The Peripheral Nervous System

The **Peripheral Nervous System** consists of the nerves that branch out from the *Central Nervous System* and connect it to other body parts. It includes twelve pairs of *cranial nerves* which arise from the under-surface of the brain, and thirty-one pairs of *spinal nerves* connected to the spinal cord. For a listing of those peripheral nerves, which might be of concern to the massage therapist, please see the Endangerment Site Listing found in the massage section. This portion is also subdivided into two divisions: the *Somatic System* and the *Autonomic System*.

1) Somatic System - Consists of *motor neurons* that are under *voluntary* control and connect the *CNS* to the *skin* and *skeletal muscles*. The site of union between a *motor neuron axon* and a muscle fiber is known as the *motor end-plate* or *neuromuscular junction*.

2) Autonomic Nervous System - Consists of *motor neurons* that are under *involuntary* control. This connects the *CNS* to *cardiac muscle, visceral (smooth muscle, organs),* and *glandular tissue.* This part of the nervous system regulates the autonomic functions of the body. Two anatomically and physiologically separate divisions compose the autonomic nervous system: the *Sympathetic (Thoracolumbar)* division and the *Para-sympathetic (Craniosacral)* division.

a) The *sympathetic* division of the autonomic nervous system functions chiefly as an *emergency system*. Under stress conditions, either physical or emotional causes, sympathetic impulses increase greatly to most *visceral effectors*. In fact, one of the very first steps in the body's complex defense mechanism against stress is a sudden and marked increase in sympathetic activity. This brings about a group of responses that all go on at the same time. Together they make the body ready to expend maximum energy and to engage in maximum physical exertion (i.e. running or fighting). Walter B. Cannon coined a descriptive and now famous phrase, the "fight or flight" syndrome. Some particularly important physiological changes for maximum energy expenditure are: faster, stronger heartbeat; dilated blood vessels in skeletal muscles; dilated bronchi; increased blood sugar levels from stimulated glycogenolysis; and the increased secretion of epinephrine. *Epinephrine* is a hormone secreted by the *adrenal medulla*. It reinforces and prolongs the effects of the neurotransmitter *norepinephrine*, which is released by most sympathetic post-ganglionic fibers.

b) The **parasympathetic** division functions under normal, everyday conditions as the main regulator of many *visceral effectors* (i.e. heart, digestive tract smooth muscle, glands that secrete digestive juices, and the endocrine gland for secretion of insulin). Ordinarily these visceral effectors receive more impulses over *cholinergic parasympathetic fibers* than they do over *adrenergic fibers*. *Acetylcholine* is the neurotransmitter of the para-sympathetic system. It stimulates the secretion of digestive juices and insulin. It also stimulates the smooth muscle of the digestive tract and thereby increases *peristalsis*. In short, the parasympathetic system functions to promote digestion and elimination.

3) Cranial Nerves and Their Functions

Twelve pairs of **cranial nerves** arise from various locations on the under surface of the brain. These nerves originate from the brain stem, with the exception of the first pair, which arises from the cerebrum. They all pass from their sites of origin through the foramen of the skull and lead to parts of the head, neck, and trunk.

The **spinal cord** is composed of ***thirty-one segments***, each giving rise to a pair of spinal nerve roots. These nerves branch out to various body parts and connect them with the central nervous system. At the level of vertebra T-12 the spinal cord tapers to a conical portion named the *conus medullaris*. This portion ends at approximately the L-1, L-2 disc. At this level, a structure known as the *filum terminale* (terminal fibers) arises. The nerve roots arising from this inferior portion are collectively known as the ***cauda equina*** (horses tail).

	Cranial Nerves	**Spinal Nerves**
Origin:	Base of Brain.	Spinal Cord
Distribution:	Mainly to head and neck.	Skin, skeletal muscles, joints, blood vessels, sweat glands, and mucosa, except of the head and neck.
Structure:	Some composed of sensory fibers only; some of both motor axons & sensory dendrites; some motor fibers belong to somatic nervous system, some to autonomic.	All of them composed of sensory dendrites and motor axons, some somatic, some autonomic.
Function:	Vision, hearing, sense of smell, sense of taste, eye movements, etc.	Sensations, movements, and sweat secretion.

Cranial Nerve		Type	Function
I	Olfactory	Sensory	Sense of smell.
II	Optic	Sensory	Vision.
III	Oculomotor	Motor	Raise eyelids, move eyes, regulate the size of pupils, focus of lenses.
IV	Trochlear	Motor	Eye movements, *proprioception*.
V	Trigeminal	Mixed	Sensations of the head and face, chewing movements, and muscle sense.
VI	Abducens	Motor	Produce movements of the eyes.
VII	Facial	Mixed	Facial expressions, secretion of saliva, taste.
VIII	Vestibulo-cochlear	Sensory	Balance or equilibrium sense. Hearing.
IX	Glosso-pharyngeal	Mixed	Taste and other sensations of tongue, swallowing, secretion of saliva, aid in reflex control of blood pressure and respiration.
X	Vagus	Mixed	Transmit impulses to muscles associated with speech, swallowing, the heart, smooth muscles of visceral organs in the thorax, and abdomen.
XI	Accessory	Motor	Turning movements of the head, Movements of the shoulder and viscera, voice production.
XII	Hypoglossal	Motor	Tongue movements.

4) General (Somatic) and Special Senses

Before parts of the nervous system can act in the control of body functions and the maintenance of homeostasis, they must be aware of what is happening inside and outside of the body. This information is gathered by *sensory receptors,* which are sensitive to environmental changes. One group of receptors is widely distributed throughout the skin and deeper tissues and is associated with the **somatic senses** of *touch, pressure, temperature,* and *pain*. The second group of receptors function as parts of complex, specialized *sensory organs* responsible for the **special senses** of *smell, taste, vision, hearing,* and *equilibrium*.

a) Types of Sensory Receptors

1) Superficial Receptors - Located in the *skin* and *mucosa*. Stimulation of them initiates sensations of *touch, pressure, heat, cold,* and *pain*.

2) Deep Receptors - Located in *muscle, tendons,* and *joints*. Stimulation of them initiates sensations of *position, vibration, deep pressure,* and *deep pain* (proprioceptors).

3) Visceral Receptors - Located in the *viscera*. Stimulation initiates such sensations as *hunger* and *visceral pain*.

4) Special Receptors - Located in the *eye, ear, mouth,* and **nose**. Stimulation initiates what we call our *special senses,* which include vision, hearing, equilibrium, taste, and smell.

5) Pain Receptors - (nociceptors) Classified according to the location of the pain receptors stimulated, either **somatic** or **visceral**. *Somatic* pain may be superficial, from stimulation of skin receptors, or it may be deep, from stimulation of receptors in the skeletal muscles, fascia, tendons, and joints. *Visceral* pain results from stimulation of receptors located in the viscera. Impulses are conducted from these receptors to the cord primarily by sensory fibers in sympathetic nerves and only rarely in parasympathetic nerves. The cerebrum does not always interpret the source of pain accurately. Sometimes it erroneously refers the pain to a surface area instead of to the region in which the stimulated receptors actually are located. This phenomenon is called **referred pain**. It occurs only as a result of stimulation of pain receptors located in *deep* structures (notably, viscera, joints, and skeletal muscles), never from stimulation of skin receptors.

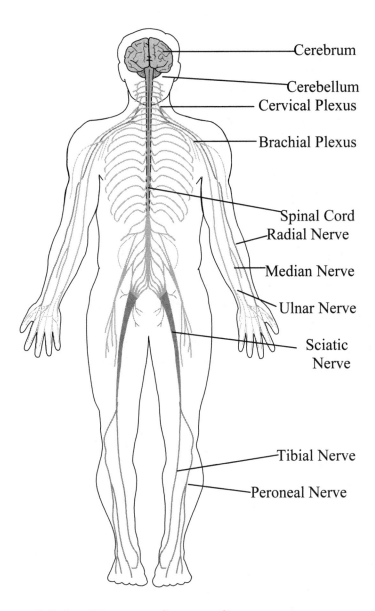

- Cerebrum
- Cerebellum
- Cervical Plexus
- Brachial Plexus
- Spinal Cord
- Radial Nerve
- Median Nerve
- Ulnar Nerve
- Sciatic Nerve
- Tibial Nerve
- Peroneal Nerve

Major Nervous System Structures

Deep somatic pain and visceral pain may be referred, but not superficial somatic pain. Pain originating in the viscera and other deep structures is generally interpreted as coming from the skin area whose sensory fibers enter the same segment of the spinal cord as the sensory fibers from the viscera. Sensory fibers from the heart enter the first to fourth thoracic segments, as do sensory fibers from the skin areas over the heart and on the inner surface of the left arm. Pain in the heart is referred to those skin areas, but the reason for this is not clear. Because stimulation of pain receptors may give warning of potentially harmful environmental changes, pain receptors are also called *nociceptors*. Any type of stimulus, provided that it is sufficiently intense, seems to be adequate for stimulating nociceptors in the skin and mucosa. In contrast, only marked changes in pressure and certain chemicals (ex: Kinins, Substance P, Serotonin) can stimulate nociceptors located in the viscera. Sometimes this knowledge proves useful. For example, it enables a physician to cauterize the cervix without giving an anesthetic, but with assurance that the patient will not suffer pain from the intense heat. On the other hand, if the intestine becomes markedly distended, as it sometimes does following surgery, the patient will experience pain. So too, will the individual whose heart becomes ischemic because of coronary occlusion. Presumably the resulting cellular oxygen deficiency leads to the formation of accumulation of chemicals that stimulate nociceptors in the heart.

4. The Endocrine System

The endocrine system consists of a variety of *glandular organs* acting together with the nervous system to control activities and maintain homeostasis. The glands of the endocrine system secrete **hormones,** which are transmitted in body fluids to the tissues they affect. The effect of the endocrine system is very slow and long lasting. As a group, endocrine glands are concerned with the regulation of metabolic processes.

a. Types of Endocrine Glands, their Locations, and Secretions

1) Pituitary Gland - Attached to the base of the brain. Consists of an anterior and posterior lobe. (The anterior lobe is housed in the *sella turcica* of the *sphenoid bone*.) The **anterior pituitary** is composed largely of epithelial cells, whereas the **posterior pituitary** consists largely of neuroglial cells, which support nerve fibers originating in the hypothalamus. (Most pituitary secretions are controlled by the *hypothalamus*) Hormones produced by the **pituitary gland**, their target tissues/organs, and actions are shown below.

Anterior Lobe		
Hormone	*Target Tissue*	*Action*
Growth Hormone (GH)	Body Cells	Stimulates increase in size and rate of body cells; enhances movement of amino acids through membranes.
Prolactin	Mammary Glands	Sustains milk production after birth.
Thyroid Stimulating Hormone (TSH)	Thyroid Gland	Controls secretion of hormones from the thyroid gland.
Adrenocorticotropic Hormone (ACTH)	Adrenal Cortex	Controls secretion of certain hormones from the adrenal cortex.
Follicle Stimulating Hormone (FSH)	Ovary; Testes	Responsible for the development of egg-containing follicles in ovaries, stimulates follicle cells to secrete estrogen; in males, stimulates the production of sperm cells.
Luteinizing Hormone (LH)	Ovary; Testes	Promotes secretion of the sex hormone testosterone in males; plays a role in the release of egg cells in females.
Melanocyte-Stimulating Hormone (MSH)	Epithelial Tissue	Stimulates the production of melanin.

Posterior Lobe		
Hormone	*Target Tissue*	*Action*
Antidiuretic Hormone (ADH)	Kidneys	Causes kidneys to reduce the excretion of water; in high concentration causes blood pressure to rise.
Oxytocin	Uterus; Mammary Glands	Causes contractions of muscles in uterus wall; causes muscles in milk ducts to contract.

2) Thyroid Gland - Located in the neck, just below the larynx on either side and in front of the trachea. It has a special ability to remove iodine from the blood. Consists of many hollow secretory parts called *follicles*. Hormones secreted by the thyroid gland, their target tissues/organs, and actions are shown below.

Thyroid Gland		
Hormones	*Target Tissue*	*Action*
Thyroxine (T4)	Body Cells	Increases rate of energy release from carbohydrates; increases rate of protein synthesis; accelerates growth; stimulates activity in the nervous system. (i.e. increases cell metabolism of most of the cells of the body)
Triiodothyronine (T3)	Body Cells	Same as above, but more powerful.
Calcitonin	Osteocytes	Decreases blood calcium level by inhibiting the release of calcium from bones.

3) Parathyroid Glands - Located on the posterior surface of the thyroid. Consists of secretory cells that are closely associated with capillaries. Hormones produced by the **parathyroid glands**, their target tissues/organs, and actions are as follows:

Parathyroid Glands		
Hormones	*Target Tissue*	*Action*
Parathyroid Hormone (PTH)	Bones, Intestines, Kidneys	Stimulates the release of calcium from bone, conservation of calcium by the kidneys, and absorption of calcium by the intestines. The resulting increase in blood calcium level inhibits the secretion of this hormone.

4) Adrenal Glands - Located on top of the kidneys. Each gland consists of a *medulla* and a *cortex*. These glands are composed of closely packed masses of epithelial cells and are very vascular. Hormones produced, their target tissues/organs, and actions are shown below:

Adrenal Medulla		
Hormones	*Target Tissue*	*Action*
Epinephrine	Sympathetic Nervous System	Causes increase in heart rate, rise in blood pressure, rise in blood glucose, increase in breathing rate, dilation of airways, and decrease in digestive activities.
Norepinephrine	Same as above	Same as above.

Adrenal Cortex		
Hormones	*Target Tissue*	*Action*
Aldosterone	Kidneys	Causes the kidneys to conserve sodium ions and excrete potassium ions. Promotes water conservation by reducing urine output.
Cortisol	Body Cells	Influences the metabolism of carbohydrates, proteins and fats; decreases the permeability of capillary walls to reduce inflammatory response.
Estrogen	In Female	Stimulates development of female secondary sexual characteristics.
Testosterone	In Male	Male hormone from interstitial cells of testes.

5) Pineal Gland - Located between the cerebral hemispheres on the roof of the third ventricle. Stimulated by light. Hormone released is shown below.

Pineal Gland		
Hormone	*Target Tissue*	*Action*
Melatonin	Body Cells	Produced by response to light. Increases at night and decreases during the day. May be involved in the regulation of some *circadian (24 hour) & seasonal rhythms*.

6) Pancreas - Located in back of the stomach and behind the parietal peritoneum. The *endocrine* portion consists of cells arranged in clusters closely associated with blood vessels. This group of cells, called the *Islets of Langerhans*, includes two distinct types of cells, **alpha cells** and **beta cells**. Hormones produced, target tissues/organs, and actions shown below:

Pancreas		
Hormones	*Target Tissue*	*Action*
Glucagon (Alpha Cells)	Liver	Stimulates the liver to convert glycogen into glucose, causing the blood glucose level to rise.
Insulin (Beta Cells)	Body Cells	Promotes the movement of glucose through cell membranes, causing the blood glucose level to fall; stimulates the liver to convert glucose into glycogen; promotes the transport of amino acids into cells; enhances the synthesis of proteins and fats.

7) Thymus - Located in the mediastinum, behind the sternum and between the lungs. Diminishes in size with age. Hormone secreted is shown below:

Thymus		
Hormone	*Target Tissue*	*Action*
Thymosin	Blood	Increases the production of white blood cells to increase immune function.

8) Reproductive Glands - Located in the pelvic cavity. Includes the *ovaries, testes, and placenta*.

Ovaries - located in the pelvic cavity.	Secretes *estrogen & progesterone*.
Testes - located in the scrotum.	Secretes *testosterone*.
Placenta - located in the uterine wall.	Secretes *estrogen, progesterone,* and *gonadotropin*.

5. The Blood

Blood is a type of connective tissue whose cells are suspended in a liquid intercellular matrix called ***plasma***. It functions to transport oxygen from respiratory organs and nutrients from the digestive system to the body cells. It then carries wastes from these cells to the respiratory and excretory organs. It transports hormones from the endocrine glands to *target* tissues and bathes the body cells in a liquid whose composition is relatively stable. Blood also aids in temperature control by distributing heat from skeletal muscles and other active organs to all body parts. The *blood, heart,* and *blood vessels* constitute the ***circulatory system***.

The human body contains approximately five quarts of blood. ***Plasma***, the fluid portion of blood, is one of the three major body fluids. (*Interstitial* and *intracellular* fluids are the other two.) Plasma makes up about 55% of the blood volume. Ninety-one percent of this volume is water, with the remaining 9% consisting of nutrients (i.e. proteins, fats, and carbohydrates), gases, chemicals, electrolytes, and hormones. The blood cells are suspended in the plasma. The term ***formed elements*** is used to designate the various kinds of blood cells collectively. This constitutes about 45% of the blood. The three types of blood cells are: ***red blood cells (erythrocytes); white blood cells (leukocytes);*** and ***platelets (thrombocytes)***.

a) Red Blood Cells (Erythrocytes) - Formed in the red marrow of bones. Tiny, biconcave disks whose shapes provide increased surface area through which gases can diffuse. Each red blood cell is about one-third ***hemoglobin*** by volume, and this substance is responsible for the color of the blood. Their shape allows for easy passage through capillaries. Function in the transportation of oxygen and carbon dioxide. Their life span is 105-120 days. They are destroyed by reticuloendothelial cells in the lining of blood vessels in the liver, spleen, and bone marrow by *phagocytosis*.

b) White Blood Cells (Leukocytes) - *Granular leukocytes* are formed in red marrow. Some lymphocytes later migrate to the liver and thymus. They function in the body's defense against invasion by microorganisms, some by phagocytosis of foreign particles, others produce antibodies of immunity. Leukocytes may be stimulated by the presence of chemicals released by damaged cells and move toward these chemicals. **Basophils** release *heparin*, which inhibits blood clotting. **Eosinophils** act to detoxify foreign proteins that enter the body through the lungs or intestinal tract. They may also release enzymes that cause blood clots to break down. The life span of a white blood cell is not definitely known. Probably some are destroyed by phagocytosis.

c) Platelets (Thrombocytes) - Formed in red marrow. Function to initiate clotting to maintain homeostasis. Their life span & means of destruction are unknown.

6. The Cardiovascular System

The **cardiovascular system** is the portion of the circulatory system that includes the **heart** and **blood vessels**. It functions to move blood between body cells and the various organs that are connected with the external environment. The heart acts as a pump that forces blood through the blood vessels, which form a closed system of ducts that transports blood and allows for the exchanges of gases, nutrients, and wastes between the blood and the body cells.

a. Anatomy of the Cardiovascular System

1) Heart - Located within the mediastinum just behind the body of the sternum with the lower border *(apex)* lying on the diaphragm. Approximately two thirds is to the left of the midline of the body and one third is to the right. Posteriorly the heart rests on the bodies of the fifth through the eighth thoracic vertebrae. This four-chambered muscular organ is divided into two **atria** and two **ventricles** and functions as two pumps. The *right atrium* receives blood from the *vena cavae* and *coronary sinus*. The *right ventricle* pumps deoxygenated blood through the *pulmonary arteries* where it is oxygenated in the lungs and returns to the *left atrium* through the *pulmonary veins*. The *left ventricle* pumps blood into the *aorta* whose branches distribute blood to all parts of the body. Four sets of valves are of importance to the normal flow of blood through the heart carrying it in one direction only. Two of these, the **atrioventricular valves**, are located between the atria and ventricles; the *tricuspid valve* (consisting of three flaps of endocardium) on the right and the *bicuspid or mitral valve* (consisting of two flaps of endocardium) on the left. The other two, the **semilunar valves**, are located inside the pulmonary artery - arising from the right ventricle, and the aorta - arising from the left ventricle. The muscular tissue of the heart, **myocardium**, is *striated* and under *involuntary* control.

2) Blood Vessels - There are three kinds of blood vessels: **arteries, veins,** and **capillaries**. Although no vessels are unimportant, several may be of particular interest to the massage therapist because of their relatively vulnerable location (i.e. the vertebral arteries move toward the head through the transverse foramen and are thus susceptible to trauma during extreme rotation of the cervical spine). Please see the Endangerment Site Listing found in the massage section.

    a) Arteries - Composed primarily of muscular and elastic tissue with a connective tissue covering. These strong vessels carry blood *away* from the heart and can withstand great pressure from the heart pump. All arteries, except the pulmonary artery and its branches, carry oxygenated blood. Pulmonary arteries carry deoxygenated blood from the right ventricle to the lungs for oxygenation. *(the Aorta is the largest artery)*

    b) Arterioles - Small arteries, carry blood from the artery to the capillaries. A partial cuff of smooth muscle on the arteriole, *precapillary sphincter*, controls blood flow to the capillaries and is of great importance for maintaining normal blood pressure and circulation.

    c) Veins - Composed largely of connective tissue with some muscular and elastic tissue. Contain *valves*, which prevent the backflow of blood and aid returning blood back to the heart. Veins function to carry blood *toward* the heart and are subjected to less pressure than arteries. All veins, except the pulmonary veins, contain deoxygenated blood. Pulmonary veins carry oxygenated blood from the lungs to the left atrium. Small veins are known as *venules*. **Note:** Both arteries and veins are macroscopic structures. *(the Great Saphenous is the longest vein)*

    d) Capillaries - Microscopic vessels that are only one cell thick, making them very permeable and providing for diffusion and osmosis to and from tissues. Function is to carry blood from arterioles to venules.

3) Circulation is defined as the blood flow through a closed circuit of vessels. Below are the major circulatory routes:

    a) Systemic Circulation - Blood flow from the left ventricle into the aorta, through arteries, arterioles, capillaries, venules, and veins to all parts of the body and returning to the right atrium of the heart.

    b) Pulmonary Circulation - Blood flow from the right ventricle through pulmonary arteries into lung arterioles, capillaries, and venules, returning to the left atrium through pulmonary veins.

    c) Coronary Circulation - Blood flow from the aorta back to the heart muscle (myocardium) through coronary arteries.

d) Hepatic Portal Circulation - Veins from the organs of digestion, the spleen, stomach, pancreas, gallbladder, and intestines, send their blood to the liver by means of the hepatic portal vein. Here the blood mixes with arterial blood in the capillaries and is drained from the liver by the hepatic portal veins which join the inferior vena cava.

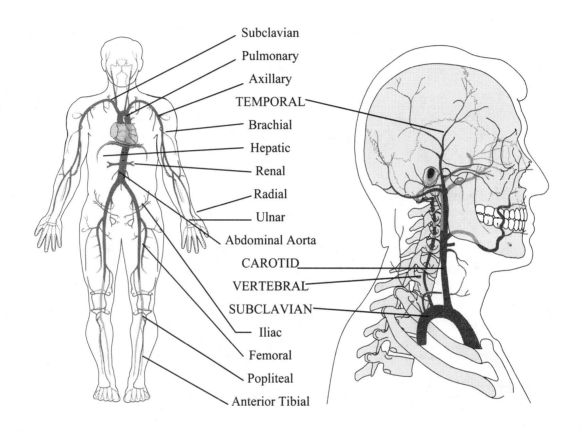

Main Arteries of the Body, Head, and Neck

(Note that the vertebral arteries pass through the transverse foramen of the cervical vertebrae)

b. Physiology of the Cardiovascular System

The cardiovascular system functions in the control of circulation throughout the body. Its control mechanisms not only *maintain* circulation, but *vary* it as well. (i.e. increase blood flow per minute when activity increases and decrease blood flow when activity decreases.) Blood circulates because a blood pressure gradient exists within its vessels. This is the primary principle of circulation. The primary determinant of arterial pressure is the volume of blood in the arteries.

1) Blood Pressure - The force exerted by the blood against the inner walls of blood vessels. This term is most commonly used to refer to the pressure within arteries. Arterial blood pressure is clinically measured with a *sphygmomanometer*. The maximum pressure achieved in ventricular contraction is called the **systolic pressure**. When the ventricles relax, the arterial pressure drops, and the amount that remains in the arteries is termed the **diastolic pressure**. Normal range for systolic pressure is about 120 to 140 millimeters of mercury (mm. Hg.), and normal range of diastolic pressure is about 80 to 90 mm. Hg. Factors that determine blood pressure would include: blood volume, heart rate, blood viscosity, elasticity of the vessels, and the strength of the heartbeat. Blood pressure is highest as the blood exits the heart, decreasing greatly in the capillary beds, and is almost non-existent in larger veins.

2) Pulse - Alternate expanding and recoiling of an arterial wall can be felt as a pulse. This is caused by the intermittent injections of blood from the heart into the aorta with each ventricular contraction. A pulse can be felt because of the elasticity of arterial walls.

7. The Lymphatic System

During the exchange of fluids, nutrients, gases, and wastes between the blood and body tissues, more fluid leaves the capillaries than returns to them. The lymphatic system provides pathways through which this tissue fluid can be transported as lymph from the interstitial spaces to veins, where it becomes part of the blood and is returned to the right atrium of the heart by the vena cavae. The lymphatic system also helps to defend the tissues against infections by filtering particles from the lymph, and producing lymphocytes, a type of white blood cell, which is vital in our role against invasion by microorganisms.

a. Anatomy & Physiology of the Lymphatic System

1) Lymph - The interstitial fluid composed of water, electrolytes, sugars and maybe proteins, which leaked out of capillaries into tissue spaces. Once this fluid is **inside** the *lymphatic capillary* it is known as lymph.

2) Lymphatic Capillaries - Microscopic, closed-ended tubes that extend into the interstitial spaces of most body tissues. Consist of a single layer of squamous epithelial cells.

3) Lymphatic Vessels - A merging of lymphatic capillaries into a larger vessel. Like veins, lymphatic vessels contain *valves*, which help to prevent the back flow of lymph. Lymphatic vessels lead to specialized organs called **lymph nodes**. (The largest and most proximal lymphatic vessels are the *Right Lymphatic Duct* - drains upper right quadrant of body and the *Thoracic Duct* - drains the remaining three quadrants of body).

4) Lymph Nodes - A mass of lymphoid tissue located along the course of a lymphatic vessel. These nodes function in *hemopoiesis*; the lymphatic tissue of lymph nodes forms **lymphocytes** and **monocytes**, the non-granular white blood cells and plasma cells. Lymphocytes act against foreign particles, such as bacterial cells and viruses, which are carried to the lymph nodes by the lymphatic vessels. Lymph nodes also contain various kinds of phagocytic cells, which act to engulf and destroy worn out cells, foreign substances, and cellular debris. In this manner, the lymph nodes help defend the body against microorganisms that have gained entrance into the tissues, and the filtration of foreign particles and cellular debris from lymph before it is returned to the bloodstream. The structure of the sinus channels within the lymph nodes slows the lymph flow through them. This process gives the reticuloendothelial cells that line the channels time to remove microorganisms and other injurious particles, cancer cells and soot, for example, from the lymph and phagocytose them. Sometimes, however, such hordes of microorganisms enter the nodes that the phagocytes cannot destroy enough of them; **adentitis**, then, results. Also, because cancer cells often break away from a malignant tumor and enter lymphatics, they travel to the lymph nodes, where they may set up new growths. This may inhibit the return of lymph to the blood. For example, if tumors block axillary node channels, fluid accumulates in the interstitial spaces of the arm, causing the arm to markedly swell. **Tonsils** are partially encapsulated lymph nodules located in the **pharynx**. Two lymphatic organs whose functions are closely related to those of the lymph nodes are the **thymus** and **spleen**.

Locations of Lymph Nodes

    a) Submental & Submaxillary Groups - Located in the floor of the mouth. Lymph from the nose, lips, and teeth drain through these nodes.

    b) Superficial Cervical Glands - Located along the lower border of the mandible, in the neck along the sternocleidomastoid muscle, and deep within the neck along the paths of the larger blood vessels. These nodes drain the skin of the scalp and face, tissues of the nasal cavity and pharynx, lymph from the head (which has already passed through other nodes), and neck.

    c) Superficial Cubital or Supratrochlear Nodes - Located just above the bend of the elbow. Lymph from the forearm passes through these nodes.

    d) Axillary Nodes - Twenty to 30 large nodes clustered deep within the underarm and upper chest regions. Lymph from the arm and upper part of the thoracic wall, including the breast, drains through these nodes.

e) **Inguinal Nodes** - Located in the groin. Drain lymph from the legs, external genitalia, and the lower abdominal wall.

f) **Pelvic Cavity** - Located in the pelvic cavity primarily along the paths of the iliac blood vessels. They receive lymph from the lymphatic vessels of the pelvic viscera.

g) **Abdominal Cavity** - Occur along the main branches of the mesenteric arteries and the abdominal aorta. Drain the abdominal viscera.

h) **Thoracic Cavity** - Located within the mediastinum and along the trachea and bronchi. They receive lymph from the thoracic viscera and from the internal wall of the thorax.

5) **Thymus** - A soft, bi-lobed structure whose lobes are surrounded by capsules of connective tissue. Located within the mediastinum, in front of the aorta and behind the upper part of the sternum. Produces hormones to enhance the functions of the immune system.

6) **Spleen** - Largest of the lymphatic organs. Located in the upper left portion of the abdominal cavity, just beneath the diaphragm and behind the stomach. The chambers of the spleen are filled with *blood* instead of lymph. Functions as a *blood reservoir*.

8. The Respiratory System

Before the body cells can utilize nutrients such as glucose, triglycerides, and amino acids, they must be supplied with oxygen. The respiratory system functions to obtain oxygen, release carbon dioxide, filter incoming air, control the temperature and water content of incoming air, produce sound, and play roles in the sense of smell and the regulation of (tissue & blood) pH.

a. Anatomy of the Respiratory System - The *organs* of the respiratory system include the *nose, pharynx, larynx, trachea, bronchi, alveoli,* and *lungs.* Together they constitute the lifeline, the air supply line of the body. We shall first describe the structure and functions of these organs and then discuss the physiology of the respiratory system as a whole.

1) **Nose** - A part of the face supported by bone and cartilage. The space behind the nose, the *nasal cavity*, is lined with mucous membranes capable of warming, moistening, and filtering incoming air. The *sinuses* are spaces in the bones of the skull that open into the nasal cavity, also lined with mucous membrane continuous with that of the nasal cavity.

2) Pharynx - or *throat*. Located behind the mouth and between the nasal cavity and *larynx*. Functions as a common passage for air & food. Aids in producing vocal sounds.

3) Larynx - An enlargement at the top of the trachea. Serves as a passageway for air and helps prevent foreign objects from entering the trachea. Composed of muscles and cartilages. Contains the vocal cords, which produce sounds by vibrating as air passes over them.

4) Trachea - W*indpipe*. Extends into the thoracic cavity in front of the esophagus where it splits into right and left *bronchi*. The inner wall is lined with ciliated mucous membrane, which continues to filter incoming air and move entrapped particles upward to the pharynx. Within the tracheal wall are about twenty C-shaped rings of *hyaline cartilage,* which prevents the trachea from collapsing and blocking the airway.

5) Bronchi - Consists of the branched airways that lead from the trachea to the air sacs. Their walls contain incomplete cartilaginous rings. Functions to distribute air to all parts of the lungs. They continue to branch and form small *bronchioles*, which do not contain these rings. At the very ends of the finest tubes are located the *alveoli.*

6) Alveoli - Microscopic air sacs located at the distal ends of bronchioles. They are a single cell thick and are lined with liquid *surfactant,* which serves to hold open the delicate alveoli. Functions to allow for the exchange of gases between the air and blood.

7) Lungs - Right and left lungs. Separated by the mediastinum and enclosed by the diaphragm and thoracic cage. The right lung has three lobes, while the left lung has two. Each lobe is composed of *lobules*, which contain alveoli, blood vessels, and supporting tissues.

b. Physiology of Breathing

Inspiration and *expiration* movements are accompanied by changes in the size of the thoracic cavity. During *inspiration*, air is forced into the lungs by atmospheric pressure. Inspiration occurs when the pressure inside the thorax is reduced and the diaphragm moves downward as the thoracic cage moves upward and outward. Expansion of the lungs is aided by surface tension that holds the pleural membranes tightly together. The alveoli do not collapse due to the presence of *surfactant*, a substance produced by the lungs, which reduces surface tension. The force of *expiration* comes from the elastic recoil of tissues. This process is aided by the thoracic and abdominal wall muscles that pull the thoracic cage downward and inward to compress the abdominal organs.

The respiratory system functions as an *air distributor* and *gas exchanger* in order that oxygen may be supplied to and carbon dioxide be removed from the body's cells. Since most of our billions of cells lie too far distant from air to exchange gases directly with it, air must first exchange gases with blood, blood must circulate, and finally blood and cells must exchange gases. These events require the functioning of two systems, namely, the *respiratory system* and the *circulatory system*. All parts of the respiratory system (except its microscopic sized sacs, *alveoli*,) function as air distributors. Only the *alveoli* serve as gas exchangers.

9.   The Digestive System

Since most food substances are composed of chemicals whose molecules cannot pass through cell membranes and so cannot be absorbed by the cells, the digestive system is necessary to handle this function. Its parts are adapted to ingest foods, secrete enzymes that modify food molecules, to absorb the products of digestion and to eliminate unused residues. Digestion means literally "the breaking down of food." This occurs in two ways, *mechanical* and *chemical*. Mechanical digestion is accomplished by chewing and the contraction of visceral muscle in the hollow organs. Chemical digestion is accomplished by the enzymes that are secreted into the *alimentary canal* by the accessory organs. Movement of food materials through this system is due to muscular contractions, known as *peristalsis*, in the wall of the *alimentary canal*. This canal is contiguous with the outside world and extends from the mouth to the anus with several accessory organs that contribute secretions into the canal. These functions are controlled largely by interactions between parts of the digestive, nervous and endocrine systems. The *organs of the digestive system include: the mouth, pharynx, esophagus, stomach, small intestine, and large intestine.*

a. Anatomy & Physiology of the Digestive System

1) Mouth - First portion of the alimentary canal. Adapted to receive food, prepare it for digestion, and begin the digestion of starch. It also functions as an organ of speech and pleasure. The (chemical) digestion of carbohydrates begins in the mouth.

2) Pharynx - Its muscular walls contain fibers arranged in circular and longitudinal groups. Serves as a passageway for food to be transported to the stomach. Swallowing occurs as food is mixed with saliva and forced into the pharynx. There, involuntary reflexes move the food into the *esophagus* and then to the stomach.

3) Esophagus - Passes through the mediastinum and penetrates the diaphragm. Some circular muscular fibers at the end of the esophagus help to prevent the regurgitation of food from the stomach. Passes food matter into the stomach.

4) Stomach - A J-shaped, pouch-like organ that lies under the diaphragm in the upper left portion of the abdominal cavity. Functions to receive food from the esophagus, serve as a reservoir to store food until it can be partially digested and move farther along the gastrointestinal tract, mix food with *gastric juice* to aid in the digestion of food, initiate the digestion of proteins, carry on a limited amount of absorption, and move food into the *small intestine*. The (chemical) digestion of proteins begins in the stomach.

5) Small Intestine - Extends from the stomach to the *large intestine*. Consists of three portions: the *duodenum, jejunum,* and *ileum*. Lined with *villi* to aid in the mixing and absorption of food. Functions to complete the digestion of foods, receive digestive enzymes from the *pancreas* and bile from the *liver,* absorb the end products of digestion into blood and lymph, and transport the residues to the large intestine. The small intestine also secretes hormones that help control the secretion of pancreatic juice, bile, and intestinal juice. The (chemical) digestion of fats begins in the small intestine. The (chemical) digestion of all other nutrients is completed in the small intestine.

6) Large Intestine - Consists of longitudinal muscle fibers and the presence of fatty appendages in the serous layer. Its parts are divided into the *cecum*, colon, and *rectum*. It begins in the lower right side of the abdominal cavity, where the *ileum* joins the *cecum*. From there the large intestine leads upward on the right side (*ascending colon*), crosses obliquely to the left (*transverse colon*), descends into the pelvis (*descending colon*), and connects to the rectum by the *sigmoid colon*. At its distal end it opens to the outside of the body as the anus. The main function of the large intestine is to absorb water, electrolytes and a few vitamins (B-12 & K), secrete mucus, and eliminate the wastes of digestion.

b. The digestive system also contains several **accessory organs** that are located in the main digestive organs or open into them. They are: the *salivary glands, teeth, liver, gallbladder, pancreas,* and *vermiform appendix*.

1) Salivary Glands - Secrete *saliva,* moistens food, helps bind food particles together, begins digestion of carbohydrates, makes taste possible, and helps cleanse the mouth. These include the *parotid glands, submaxillary glands,* and *sublingual glands.*

2) Liver - Located in the upper right portion of the abdominal cavity, lying just under the diaphragm. The liver is highly vascular and is the largest gland in the body and one of the most vital organs. It functions to produce about one pint of *bile* per day to aid in digestion, store iron and vitamins A, B-12 and D, carry on a number of important steps in the metabolism of proteins, fats and carbohydrates, detoxify a variety of substances and remove them from the body fluids, and destroy worn-out red blood cells. Also helps to maintain normal blood glucose levels.

3) Gallbladder - A pear-shaped sac attached to the ventral surface of the liver. It functions to store and secrete the bile that enters it by way of the *hepatic* and *cyctic ducts*. During this time, the gallbladder concentrates bile 5 to 10 fold by reabsorbing water. Later, when digestion is going on in the stomach and intestines, the gallbladder contracts, ejecting the concentrated bile into the *duodenum*.

4) Pancreas - Extends horizontally across the posterior abdominal wall with its head on the C-shaped curve of the *duodenum* and its tail against the *spleen*. The ***acinar units*** of the pancreas secrete the digestive enzymes found in the pancreatic juice, which are capable of digesting carbohydrates, fats, proteins, and nucleic acids. Cells within the *Islets of Langerhans* function to secrete the hormone *insulin* from ***beta cells***, which decreases blood glucose levels and exerts a major control over carbohydrate metabolism. The hormone *glucagon* is secreted from pancreatic ***alpha cells***, and increases blood glucose levels. It is interesting to note that glucagon, which is produced so close to insulin, has a directly opposite effect on carbohydrate metabolism.

5) Vermiform Appendix - Projecting downward from the cecum, it is a narrow tube with a closed end. Although it has no known digestive function, it does contain lymphatic tissue, which may serve to resist infections.

As was stated previously, the two kinds of digestive changes necessary for the absorption and metabolism of food are known as *mechanical* and *chemical*. Digestion, therefore, is the sum of all the changes food undergoes in the alimentary canal. It is a necessary and preliminary step to both the ***absorption*** and ***metabolism*** of food.

a. Absorption - The passage of substances (notably digested foods, water, salts, and vitamins) through the intestinal mucosa into the blood or lymph. Macro Nutrients (proteins, fats & carbohydrates) enter the bloodstream as amino acids, fatty acids (& glycerol), and simple sugars.

b. Metabolism - All of the chemical changes that occur within cells considered together. There are two major types of metabolic processes. One type involves the build-up of larger molecules from smaller ones, while the other involves the breakdown of larger molecules into smaller ones. They are known as ***anabolism*** and ***catabolism***.

1) Anabolism - Constructive process to synthesize the substances needed for cellular growth and repair. Uses energy to build relatively small molecules up into larger molecules. For example, simple sugar molecules of glucose are joined together by liver and muscle cells to form a larger storage form of carbohydrate molecule *(glycogen),* and amino acids are joined together to form proteins. Other molecules also joined together to form larger ones including enzymes, hormones, and antibodies. Sugars may be anabolized by the liver to form fats.

 2) Catabolism - Decomposition process in which relatively large food molecules break down to yield smaller molecules and energy. An example of this process is *digestion.* Carbohydrates are broken down into monosaccharides & disaccharides, fats into glycerol & fatty acids, and proteins into amino acids. Both fatty acids and amino acids may be further catabolised by the liver to form glucose. Simple sugars (glucose, fructose & galactose) are ultimately catabolised to form ATP.

Macronutrients (proteins, fats, & carbohydrates) supply the body with raw materials for both types of metabolic processes. Dietary proteins and their breakdown products (amino acids) are primarily used for building (anabolic) processes. Dietary fats are used in the building process, but also as energy sources. Carbohydrates are primarily used in energy producing (catabolic) processes. Micronutrients (vitamins & minerals) are primarily used as co-factors in the metabolism of the macronutrients or in the formation of enzymes, hormones, neurotransmitters, and other macromolecules. Water and food fibers (although technically considered non-nutrients) are necessary to help move food efficiently though the digestive system.

Below are tables listing the amino acids, vitamins, and minerals.

Essential Amino Acids	Nonessential Amino Acids
Isoleucine	Alanine
Leucine	Arginine
Lysine	Asparagine
Methionine	Aspartic Acid
Phenylalanine	Cysteine
Threonine	Glutamic Acid
Tryptophan	Glutamine
Valine	Glycine
	Proline
Histidine (in infants)	Serine
	Tyrosine

Fat Soluble Vitamins

Vitamin	Function	Food Source	Deficiency
A	Necessary for epithelial cell health, antioxidant	Fish oil, liver, milk, beta carotene in vegetables	Night blindness, skin disorders, increased infections
D	Essential for absorption of calcium & phosphorous	Sunlight, fish liver oils, egg yolk, & fortified milk	Rickets, Osteomalacia, Osteoporosis
E	Inhibits catabolism of certain fatty acids that help for DNA, RNA, and RBC's	Fresh nuts, wheat germ, seed oils & green leafy vegetables	Free-radical damage to cells, hemolytic anemia, nerve disorders
K	Necessary for clotting factors	Spinach, cauliflower, cabbage & liver	Delayed clotting time

Water Soluble Vitamins

Vitamin	Function	Food Source	Deficiency
B-1 Thiamine	Coenzyme in carbohydrate metabolism	Whole grains, eggs, pork, nuts, liver, & yeast	Beriberi, Neuropathy
B-2 Riboflavin	Coenzyme in carbohydrate & protein metabolism	Yeast, red meats, eggs, beets, whole grains, asparagus	Optic disorders, anemia, dermatitis
B-3 Niacin	Coenzyme in fat metabolism	Yeast, whole grains, meats, nuts, legumes	Pellagra, weakness, neuropathy, anorexia
B-6 Pyridoxine	Coenzyme in amino acid metabolism	Salmon, yeast, tomatoes, wheat, yellow corn, yogurt	Dermatitis of eyes, nose & mouth
B-12 Cyanocobalamin	Coenzyme in RBC formation	Liver, kidney, milk, eggs, cheese, & meat	Pernicious Anemia, neurological disorders
Biotin	Coenzyme in fatty acid metabolism	Yeast, liver, egg yolk, kidneys	Mental depression, pain, dermatitis
C	Collagen synthesis, wound healing, antioxidant	Citrus fruit, tomatoes, green vegetables	Scurvy, anemia, poor wound healing, infections
Folic Acid	RBC's & WBC's, developing nervous system	Green leafy vegetables, broccoli, breads, dried beans	Abnormal RBC's, neural defects in newborns
Pantothenic Acid	Conversion of lipids & amino acids into glucose	Liver, Kidney, yeast, cereal, green vegetables	Fatigue, muscle spasms, insomnia, vomiting

Mineral	Function	Food Source	Deficiency
Calcium	Bone formation, neuro-muscular function, blood clotting	Milk, egg yolk, shellfish, green leafy vegetables	Rickets, Osteoporosis, Osteomalacia, muscle disorders
Phosphorus	Bone formation, neuro-muscular function	Dairy products, meat, fish, poultry, & nuts	Bone disease, malabsorption syndromes
Potassium	Neuro-muscular function	Meats, fish, poultry, fruits, & nuts	Muscle cramps, arrhythmia
Sulfur	Cofactor in ATP production, protein structure	Beef, liver, lamb, fish, poultry, eggs, cheese, beans	Kidney stones
Sodium	Neuro-muscular function, controls fluid balance	Table salt, soy sauce, processed foods	Muscle cramps, arrhythmia, electrolyte imbalance
Chloride	Acid-base & fluid-electrolyte balance, HCL in stomach acid	Table salt, soy sauce, processed foods	Alkalosis
Magnesium	Bone formation, muscle contractions	Grains, nuts, soy, seafood, legumes	Tremors, spasms
Iron	Hemoglobin synthesis	Liver, meat, eggs, whole grains, dark green vegetables	Anemia
Iodide	Thyroid hormone	Iodized salt, seafood	Goiter, Thyroid disorders
Manganese	Coenzyme in metabolism	Whole grains, legumes, leafy vegetables	Diabetes, protein-energy disorders
Copper	Hemoglobin synthesis	Liver, meat, seafood, grains	Malabsorption, Wilson's Disease
Cobalt	Vitamin B-12 constituent	Liver, kidney, milk, eggs, cheese, & meat	Anemia (vitamin B-12 deficiency)
Zinc	Coenzyme in many processes	Seafood, oysters, meat, diary, grains	Impaired taste, smell, & wound healing
Fluoride	Hardens bones & teeth	Fish, tea, fluoridated water	Osteoporosis, dental caries
Selenium	Antioxidant, cofactor & component of teeth	Seafood, legumes, whole grains, dairy, vegetables	Dental problems
Chromium	Cofactor in glucose metabolism	Cereals, whole grains, yeast, animal protein	Poor glucose metabolism

10. The Urinary System

Since cells form a variety of waste substances as by-products of metabolic processes, the urinary system is necessary to remove these wastes so they do not accumulate in the tissues and produce a toxic effect on the body. In addition to removing wastes from the blood, the urinary system helps to maintain the normal concentrations of water and electrolytes within the body fluids. It also helps to regulate the volume of body fluids and aids in the control of blood pressure and pH. The urinary system consists of the *kidneys, ureters, urinary bladder,* and *urethra.*

a. Anatomy and Physiology of the Urinary System

1) Kidneys - A pair of glandular organs located on either side of the vertebral column, high on the posterior wall of the abdominal cavity. They are *retroperitoneal,* behind the parietal peritoneum and against the deep muscles of the back. The kidneys extend from the level of the last thoracic vertebrae to the third lumbar vertebrae. They function to remove wastes from the blood, regulate water & electrolyte concentrations, and form urine. They do so by the process of filtration, secretion and reabsorption.

2) Ureters - Muscular tubes that carry urine from the kidneys to the urinary bladder.

3) Urinary Bladder - A muscular bag located directly behind the *symphysis pubis.* It lies below the parietal peritoneum, which covers only its superior surface. Functions to store urine and forces it into the urethra.

4) Urethra - Tube leading from the urinary bladder to the outside of the body. Functions to convey urine from the bladder to the outside. Urine consists of uric acid, urea, water, and ammonia. It may contain trace amounts of amino acids and some electrolytes, depending upon the dietary intake. Urine should not contain any amount of blood or sugars.

G. Kinesiology, Biomechanics, and Gait

Muscles make bones and joints move. The nearly 700 skeletal muscles comprise up to 40-50% of the adult human body (by weight), and function to provide humans with movement, heat production, and posture.

1. Muscle Fiber Patterns - Fibers within skeletal muscle form patterns, which are visible to the naked eye. When the fibers are aligned, such as in the abdominal muscles, the pattern is described as parallel or **strap**-like (quadratus lumborum & rectus abdominis). Where the fibers run obliquely to the direction of force, the muscle is described as either **triangular** or **pennate**. If the muscle fibers insert diagonally into a tendon that runs the entire length of the muscle, the muscle is described as pennate. **Bipennate** muscles (rectus femoris) have their fibers inserting obliquely on both sides of the tendon. In **fusiform** muscles (biceps brachii), the fibers may be nearly parallel in the belly, yet converge to fuse at a tendon at one or both ends. **Multipennate** muscles (deltoid) have multiple oblique fiber directions. Some muscles have a **spiral** or twisted arrangement (latissimus dorsi).

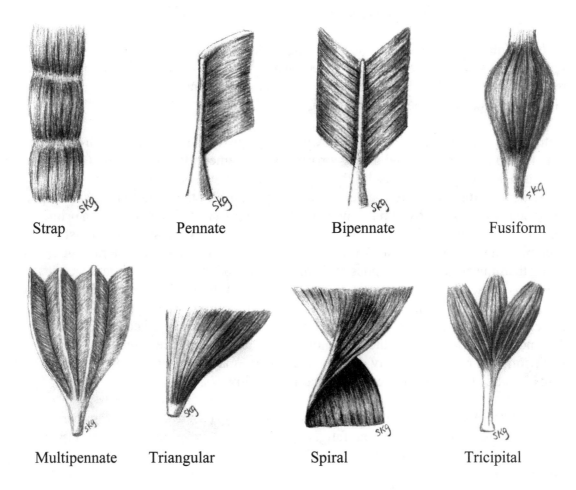

| Strap | Pennate | Bipennate | Fusiform |

| Multipennate | Triangular | Spiral | Tricipital |

2. Action of Muscles - The action of a muscle is defined as the movement that takes place when that muscle contracts. In this context, contraction is equated to shortening and relaxation is equated to lengthening. Contraction may be considered as an attempt on the part of the muscle to bring its attachments closer together. The success of a muscle to accomplish this task depends upon a number of factors including gravity, inertia, external loads, opposing muscles, and forces generated by the elastic and viscous properties of associated structures. Depending on circumstances, increasing muscle tension may result in shortening, lengthening, or maintaining its original dimensions. The three major types of muscle contractions are **isotonic**, **tonic**, and **isometric**.

   a. Isotonic contractions result in a change of the active muscle length
   Concentric isotonic contractions result in the shortening of the active muscle - positive work (up-phase of a bicep curl)
   Eccentric isotonic contractions occur as there is lengthening of the active muscle - negative work (controlled, down-phase of a bicep curl)

   b. Tonic contractions involve increased muscle tension, but do not change the active muscle length and are used to maintain position or posture

   c. Isometric (static) contractions involve increased tension in the active muscle, but overpowering external forces prevent movement

3. Kinesiology (Greek. *kinesis*, motion + *logos*, science) as defined by Thompson and Floyd, is the study or science of movement, which includes anatomical (structural) and biomechanical (mechanical) aspects of movement. The sciences of kinesiology and biomechanics employ specific terminology.

Natural movements are accomplished by using groups of muscles. Muscles are classified with regard to the role played during a particular movement. **Prime movers** (agonists) are characterized as those muscles that consistently initiate and maintain a particular movement. **Antagonists** are characterized as those muscles that wholly oppose a movement or consistently initiate and maintain the opposite movement. When prime movers and antagonists contract together they act as **fixators**. Muscles that assist in accomplishing a movement are known as **synergists**. **Neutralizers** counteract the action of another muscle to prevent undesirable movements. Given different situations, a particular muscle may act as a prime mover, antagonist, fixators, synergist, or neutralizer. Muscles perform work in a variety of situations. Convention and habit dictate that the more stable (usually heavier and more proximal) attachment is referred to as the **origin**. The more mobile (usually lighter and more distal) attachment is referred to as the **insertion**. The relative mobility of bony attachments may necessitate that the use of these two terms be closely considered with regard to any given situation.

Muscle fibers have different characteristics. *Fast-Twitch* (white - anaerobic) fibers contract rapidly and forcefully, but fatigue quickly. *Slow-Twitch* (red - aerobic) fibers contract more slowly, with less intensity, but have more endurance (& myoglobin). *Intermediate* (mixed) fibers have some characteristics of both. Genetics determine type.

4. Biomechanics - Biomechanics (Greek. *bios*, life + *mechane*, machine) is the study of mechanical laws and their application to living organisms, especially the human body and its locomotor system. Movement is brought about by the action of muscle upon rigid skeletal components or levers. Levers are rigid bars that turn about an axis or fulcrum. A fulcrum is a stable point on which a lever turns. Force is the product of mass times acceleration and either pushes or pulls on an object in an attempt to affect shape or motion. Effort is the force applied to a lever. Acceleration refers to the rate of change in speed of movement. Resistance is the opposition to a force (in some cases, weight or mass). Inertia is the reluctance of matter to change its sate of motion. Muscles supply the necessary force in biomechanics. Bones provide the mechanical advantage (levers) by which work may be accomplished. Joints form the pivotal point of movement (fulcrum) around which the levers move. By changing the location of the fulcrum with regard to the force or effort (muscle) and resistance (weight), it is possible to move heavier loads and to alter both the rate and the distance over which the load can be moved.

There are three classes of levers:

In **class I** levers, the fulcrum is located between the point at which the force is applied and the weight that is to be moved. A teeter-totter is a common example of a class I lever. In the human body, this type of lever is involved in extending the elbow against resistance.

In **class II** levers, the weight to be moved is located between the fulcrum and the point of force. A wheelbarrow typifies this type of lever. In the human body, this type of lever is involved in rising up onto the toes via plantar flexion. There are relatively few occurrences of class II levers in the human body.

In **class III** levers, the weight is on one end, the fulcrum at the other, and the force is applied between them. The lifting of a shovel utilizes this type of lever. Class III levers are the most common type in the human body. One example is flexion of the elbow.

In the human body, class I levers provide for increased range of motion, with a reduction in available strength. Class II levers provide for increased strength with a reduction of range of motion. Class III levers provide for an increase in range of motion, but with a reduction of available strength.

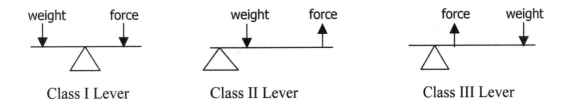

Class I Lever   Class II Lever   Class III Lever

5. Planes of Motion and Axes of Rotation - A plane of motion is an imaginary two-dimensional surface through which a limb or body segment is moved. There are three specific planes of motion in which joint movements are classified. They include the **saggittal** (anterior/posterior), **frontal** (lateral), and the **transverse** (horizontal) planes. The additional, **diagonal** (oblique) plane is a combination of more than one plane. When movement occurs in a specific plane, the involved joint(s) move or turn on an axis, which has a 90° relationship to that plane. The corresponding axes of rotation are the **lateral**, **anterioposterior**, and **vertical**. Flexion and extension movements occur in the saggittal plane. Abduction and adduction (and lateral flexion) movements occur in the frontal plane. Rotational movements (pronation and supination) movements occur in the transverse plane. Complex compound movements generally occur in the diagonal plane.

Plane	Axis	Movement
Saggittal	Lateral	Flexion/Extension
Frontal	Anterioposterior	Abduction/Adduction
Transverse	Vertical	Pronation/Supination

The **kinetic chain concept** is used to describe the complex movements of human extremities. Each bony segment of the extremity is represented as a "link" in the chain. When that chain is attached only at one end or "open", the movement of one link may not significantly affect the other links. When the chain is securely attached at both ends or "closed", movement of any one link certainly affects the others. Isolated knee extension, involves the concentric contractions of the quadriceps group, and demonstrates an **open kinetic chain** activity. When using a similar contractile force to rise from a seated position to standing, the movement represents a closed kinetic chain activity. Standing, walking and running are likewise **closed kinetic chain** activities. Open kinetic chain exercises are typically used for strengthening of isolated components. Closed kinetic chain activities or exercises are generally more applicable for developing functional performance.

Because maintaining standing posture involves a complex set of closed chain activities, it reflects the strength, balance, equilibrium and stability of a great number of structural and functions anatomical components. Postural assessment therefore provides an opportunity to evaluate the functional status of numerous bony structures, joints, fascia, and neuromuscular components.

6. Assessment - Postural assessment should include a methodical bilateral evaluation of at least the following functional areas: (1) Top of head, ears & atlas/axis, (2) C-6/C-7 vertebrae & AC joint level, (3) T-12 vertebra, (4) T-12 & S-1, (5) iliac crests/SI joint, (6) greater trochanter, (7) knee/patella & fibular head, (8) malleolus/ankles, (9) feet, arches & toes. Observe for horizontal bilateral symmetry, head forward posture, and locking of the knees. A full assessment will include evaluation of all major joints. Assessments or evaluations are most effective when completed in an organized fashion.

Any system for assessment should employ the distinct components of: **history**, **observation**, **palpation** and **specialized testing**. Each component should be completed in the proper sequence.

The **history** component should gather information regarding: the client's family health history, personal health history, chief complaint (specific location & nature of pain/etc., type of onset - sudden or insidious, duration & time of day/night, aggravating or ameliorating factors), work history, exercise history, other complaints, and previous therapies. A statement of the client's goals for therapy should also be obtained.

The **observation** component includes noting the client's mood, respiration, gait, and sitting & standing postures. Standing posture may be best observed with the aid of graphic devices. This could include a plumb line and or a wall grid. Standing observations should be made with the client positioned to provide anterior, posterior and lateral views. Evaluation of the areas noted above should be made. Any anterior to posterior (flexion/extension), side-to-side tilting (sidebending) & abduction/adduction, and rotational (twisting/ pronation/ supination) abnormalities should be noted. Gait and seated posture should be evaluated with the same level of awareness.

The **palpation** component should proceed from superficial to deep tissues, noting any abnormalities. Tissue texture, integrity, tone & elasticity, symmetry, temperature, and the client's response to touch provide useful information.

The **specialized testing** component may include passive ROM, active ROM, manual muscle (strength) testing, and regional orthopedic tests. These tests are primarily designed to provide information regarding specific structural and functional components of isolated anatomical areas. Other specialized tests are designed to rule out specific conditions. Each of these specialized tests requires a specific skill-set to insure proper (safe, valid & reliable) administration and interpretation.

Postural imbalances are occasionally described in terms of degrees of severity. *First degree* imbalances describe mild hypertrophy of target muscle(s) with corresponding hypotrophy of antagonistic muscle(s). Posture and movement are not efficient. *Second degree* imbalances describe moderate hypertrophy of target muscle(s) with corresponding hypotrophy of antagonistic muscle(s). Posture and movement distortions become apparent. *Third degree* imbalances describe marked hypertrophy of target muscle(s) with corresponding hypotrophy of antagonistic muscle(s). Gross dysfunction in posture and movement is demonstrated.

Some authors discuss the "staging" of postural and movement pathology.
Stage1: functional tension w/ slight limited mobility, painless myodystonia, and fatigue.
Stage 2: functional stress w/ more limited mobility, painful myodystonia, and fatigue.
Stage 3: pathological tissue changes w/ continued decreased mobility, painful myodystonia, marked functional debility, somatovisceral symptoms, and fatigue.
A keen awareness of the gravity of a client's condition will aid in treatment planning.

7. **Normal Joint Range of Motion** - Charts listing the joints, related motions, and the normal range of motion (in degrees) follow.

Joint	Motion	Degrees (normal ranges)
Cervical	Flexion	0 - 60
	Extension	0 - 75
	Lateral Flexion	0 - 45
	Rotation*	0 - 80
Shoulder	Flexion	0 - 180
	Extension	0 - 50
	Abduction	0 - 180
	Adduction	0 - 50
	Internal Rotation**	0 - 90
	External Rotation**	0 - 90
Elbow	Flexion	0 - 140
Radioulnar	Supination	0 - 80
	Pronation	0 - 80
Wrist	Flexion	0 - 60
	Extension	0 - 60
	Ulnar Deviation	0 - 30
	Radial Deviation	0 - 20
Thoracic	Flexion	0 - 50
	Rotation	0 - 30
Lumbar	Flexion	0 - 60+
	Extension	0 - 25
	Lateral Flexion	0 - 25
Hip	Flexion	0 - 100
	Extension	0 - 30
	Abduction	0 - 40
	Adduction	0 - 20
	Internal Rotation***	0 - 40
	External Rotation***	0 - 50
Knee	Flexion	0 - 150
Ankle	Dorsiflexion	0 - 20
	Plantar Flexion	0 - 40

Joint	Motion	Degrees (normal ranges)
Subtalar	Inversion	0 - 30
	Eversion	0 - 20
Metatarsophalangeal	Great Toe Dorsiflexion	0 - 50
	Great Toe Plantar Flexion	0 - 30

*   Measurements obtained with the client in a supine position and the head in a neutral position. The client's nose pointing to the ceiling is 0 degrees, neutral position.

**   Measurements obtained with the shoulder in 90 degrees of abduction.

*** Measurements obtained with the client in a supine position and the foot in a neutral position. The client's foot pointing to the ceiling is 0 degrees, neutral position.

Measurement of specific ROM (possible joint movement) is most efficiently done with the aid of a goniometer, which displays actual degrees. When no goniometer is available, bilateral symmetry of joint ROM should be observed and only variations from normal (either increased or decreased) noted. Charting notations commonly used include specific degrees (when using a *goniometer*), "WNL", pluses (+) and minuses (-), or up and down arrows. In any given joint, ROM can be measured both actively and passively. *Active* range of motion refers to a range through which the client's own muscles can move the joint. *Passive* range of motion refers to range through which an outside force (such as the therapist/examiner) can move the joint. Active ROM is often evaluated first. Passive ROM is then evaluated if the active ROM appears to be abnormal. ROM evaluations give valuable information. Differences between passive and active ROM raise assessment questions that demand further investigation. The inability for a client to move a joint through a full ROM may be due to a mechanical (structural) block, muscle weakness or injury, tendon pathology, joint pain, hypertonicty of the antagonist muscles, or neurological deficiencies. Excessive joint mobility may be due to mechanical (structural) abnormalities, associated muscle hypotonicity, or ligamentous laxity.

Specialized tests that screen specific joints (regions) include the Cervical Compression & Traction tests for cervical disc pathology, Adson Maneuver for Thoracic Outlet Syndrome, Cross-Over test for AC Joint injury, Empty Can & Hawkins-Kennedy tests for shoulder impingement, Speed's test for Bicipital tendonitis, Apley test for shoulder ROM, Tennis & Golfer's Elbow test, Tinel's sign for Carpal Tunnel Syndrome, Straight-Leg Raise test for lumbar disc protrusion, Thomas test for hypertonic Iliopsoas, Trendelenburg test for hip stability, Gapping and FABER (Patrick's) tests for SI joint dysfunction, Piriformis test for sciatic nerve impingement, Nobel & Ober test for Iliotibial band tightness, Clarke's sign for Patellar chondromalacia, Apley Compression test for meniscal damage, Valgus & Varus Stress tests for collateral ligament (knee) injury, Anterior and Posterior Drawer tests for ACL & PCL injury, Ankle Drawer test for ankle stability, and Thompson test for Achilles tendon rupture.

Factors such as age, systemic disease, ergonomics, postural habits, lifestyle, heredity, hydration, and nutritional status influence musculoskeletal health and performance.

8. Gait - Gait (old Norse. *geta*, a way) is defined as the manner or style of walking, including rhythm, cadence and speed.

A ***gait cycle*** is described as being the period in which a complete sequence of events takes place, beginning with the heel of one foot striking the floor and ending with the heel of the other foot striking the floor. The gait cycle is divided into two categories of events: the *stance phase* and the *swing phase.* The stance phase is defined as the time period when the limb being considered is in contact with the floor. The swing phase is defined as the time period when the limb being considered is not in contact with the ground. In walking, there always exists a period of time when both feet are in contact with the ground. This portion of the gait cycle is known as *double stance.* In the average walking person, a stance phase occurs during approximately 60% of the gait cycle while the swing phase occurs during approximately 40% of the gait cycle. As the speed of walking increases, the time spent in stance phase diminishes. Running is defined, as the gait in which there exists no double stance phase (i.e. at any given time, only one foot is in contact with the ground).

In humans, gait is primarily determined by the pelvis, upper leg (thigh), lower leg and the foot. The upper body components including the trunk, head, and arms are used in locomotion to provide momentum and counterbalance.

The components of the stance phase of gait include: ***heel strike*** (hip flexed with knee & ankle in neutral), ***foot flat*** (hip flexed with knee & ankle flexed), ***midstance*** (hip, knee & ankle in neutral), ***heel-off*** (hip extended, knee in neutral & ankle dorsiflexed), and ***toe-off*** (hip in neutral with knee flexed & ankle dorsiflexed).

The components of the swing phase of gait include: ***acceleration*** (hip flexed with knee flexed & ankle in plantar flexed), ***midswing*** (hip flexed, knee flexed & ankle in neutral), ***deceleration*** (hip flexed with knee & ankle in neutral) and ***arm swing*** (contralateral arm & leg moving in the same direction in the saggittal plane -- as each shoulder girdle advances, the pelvis & lower limb of the ipsilateral side trail behind).

The *main determinants* of gait have been defined as: *pelvic rotation, pelvic tilt, knee & hip flexion, knee & ankle interaction,* and *lateral pelvic displacement.*

It is during the *midstance* phase that the *center of gravity* of the human body reaches it's highest point in the gait cycle.

Gait is influenced by additional factors such as mass (the amount of matter in a body, the physical property that produces weight), balance (the ability to control either static or dynamic equilibrium), and momentum (the quality of motion that is equal to mass times velocity). A normal gait pattern is smooth, coordinated, and rhythmic. Abnormalities in gait result from habitual/learned patterns, pain, neurological & neuromuscular disorders, muscle weakness, myodystonia, and connective tissue restrictions.

A. Traditional Chinese Medicine (TCM)

Having a written history of more than 4500 years, TCM shares many aspects with other ancient systems, such as Ayurveda, the traditional medicine of India. The *Nei Ching* or *Classic of Internal Medicine* is believed to have been written by the mythical *Yellow Emperor* about 2500 B.C., and remains the basic reference for modern TCM thought. Early western translations of TCM writings are attributed to 18th century Portuguese missionaries who had visited China. These early translations set the stage for more current developments in TCM and may well have provided the basis for modern European massage technique. TCM has slowly developed as an empirical science, combining thousands of years of observation with several complex philosophical concepts, in an attempt to explain all observed natural phenomenon. TCM anatomical, physiological, and pathophysiological hypotheses have been postulated without the benefit of dissection or other modern analytic tools. Fundamental to traditional Chinese medicine are anatomical & physiological concepts, which therefore, differ greatly from those of the west.

B. Chi, Yin/Yang, Five Element, Channel/Organ Theory & Vital Substances

Basic to TCM is the construct of the universal bio-energy known as *Chi* (Qi), which circulates throughout the body in well-defined pathways known as *channels* or *meridians*. (It should be noted, that Chi not only animates and organizes the human body, but all of the cosmos) Channels are associated with internal organs and their observed functions. Chi circulates in a very specific 24-hour cycle from channel to channel and organ to organ, animating body functions as it moves. There are 12 major organ-related channels and various extra channels, branches, and associated vessels. Specific points with observed functions are located along each channel. More than 365 points have been located and the function of each documented. Complex interrelationships exist between specific channels, organs, and points.

In TCM, health is viewed as an expression of a balance (homeostasis) of all the forces acting on and within the body. Disease or disorder is therefore viewed as disruption of that balance. Various philosophical hypotheses have influenced the development of current TCM thought. From early Taoist thinkers came the concepts of *Yin* and *Yang*. (Yin and Yang are first referenced by the *Book of Changes*, which is dated to 700 B.C.) These two opposing yet complimentary forces influence the cosmos and all found therein. These earliest of references must have arisen from peasant observations of the cyclic nature of day/night and seasonal relationships. Day corresponds to Yang and night corresponds to Yin. This relationship was further extended to include other polar relationships as light/dark, summer/winter, heaven/earth, up/down, left/right, outside/inside, male/female, etc. As the day gives way to night, so does yang surrender to yin. In even western thought, is found the belief that "it is always darkest just before the dawn." Therefore, within each opposing force is the seed of the other. This concept has come to be synonymous with and commonly recognized as the ubiquitous Yin/Yang symbol. Ying and Yang are further described as being non-absolute, in that nothing is totally Yin or totally Yang. Moreover, the opposition of Yin & Yang is relative. It is only correct to say that something is Yin or Yang relative to something else. For example, "cold" is "Yin", when compared to "Yang" which is comparatively "hot." Yin and Yang are forever present in a dynamic and constantly changing balance. In that Yin and Yang are constantly changing, they are necessarily adjusting in proportion to achieve new balance. Although Yin and Yang are opposite, they are complimentary and interdependent. One cannot exist without the other. In fact, Yin and Yang actually transform into each other in an orderly and predictable fashion. With regard to human anatomy each structure has a predominately Yin or Yang (relative) character. Below is a table of relative qualities:

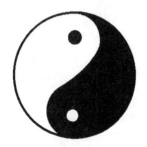

Symbol of YIN and YANG

YIN	YANG
Inferior	Superior
Interior	Exterior
Anterior	Posterior
Medial	Lateral
Structure	Function
Cooling	Warming
Wet	Dry
Quiet	Restless
Slow	Rapid
Chronic	Acute
Pale	Red
Weak	Forceful
Matter	Energy
Upward	Downward

In addition to the fundamental concepts of **Chi** and **Yin/Yang,** TCM is founded upon the theory of the **Five Elements**. The concept of Five Elements is believed to have been introduced by the *"Naturalist School"* of philosophy around 300 B.C., although strong similarities to the Five Element system are found within the *Vedic Texts* of ancient India, which date from before 2000 B.C. Five Element theory was no doubt a later addition to the TCM "system" we see today. Five Element theory states that ***Wood***, ***Fire***, ***Earth,*** ***Metal,*** and ***Water***, represent (symbolize) various qualities of all natural phenomenon including: movement, the seasons, chemical composition, taste, and all other manner of cosmological manifestation. As with Yin/Yang theory, all relationships existing between the five elements are believed to be deliberate and sequential. Of the relationships between the five elements, some are described as being nourishing or controlling. It is upon these two relationships that much of the TCM current Anatomy & Physiology, Pathophysiology and Treatment theory are based. The following illustrations and chart describe Five Element relationships and correspondences.

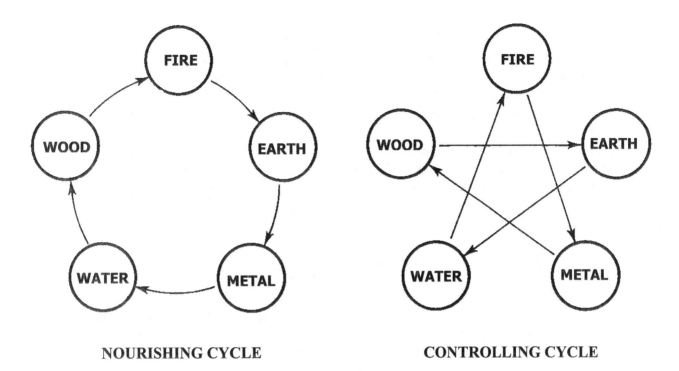

NOURISHING CYCLE　　　　　CONTROLLING CYCLE

Relationships of the Five Elements

Element:	Wood	Fire	Earth	Metal	Water
Yin Organ	Liver	Heart/Pericardium	Spleen	Lung	Kidney
Yang Organ	Gall Bladder	Small Intestine/ San Jiao	Stomach	Large Intestine	Bladder
Yin Time	1am - 3am	11am - 1pm (HT) *7pm – 9pm (PC)	9am - 11am	3am - 5am	5pm - 7pm
Yang Time	11pm - 1am	1pm - 3pm (SI) *9pm – 11pm (SJ)	7am - 9am	5am - 7am	3pm - 5pm
Color	Green	Red	Yellow	White	Blue or Black
Emotion	Anger	Joy	Worry	Grief/Sadness	Fear
Sound	Shouting	Laughing	Singing	Weeping	Groaning
Sense	Sight	Speech	Taste	Smell	Hear
Flourishes	Nails	Complexion	Lips	Body Hair	Head Hair
Nourishes	Sinews	Blood Vessels	Muscles	Skin	Bones
Flavor	Sour	Bitter	Sweet	Pungent	Salty
Season	Spring	Summer	Late Summer	Autumn	Winter

As noted in the preceding chart, all organs and channels are paired, solid organs being Yin (zang) and hollow organs being Yang (fu). The Pericardium & San Jiao are traditionally viewed as having yin & yang qualities, as participating vessels in the 24-hour flow of Chi, but only loosely associated with the Five Elements and their various relationships. All channels begin or end in the feet and hands, with Yang channels moving in an inferior direction and Yin channels moving in a superior direction. *Sunlight of heaven moves downward & water vapor of earth moves upward.* Yang channels are located on the *posterior* surface of the body and all Yin channels are found the *anterior* surface. It is very important to note that the TCM anatomical position is similar to the western model, with the exception of the hands and arms being raised overhead.

The theory of channels *(meridians, vessels)* and their collaterals is as ancient as TCM itself, with references (to the 12 regular, 8 extra, 12 divergent and various branches) being made in the *Nei Jing,* which dates to the 2nd millennium B.C. This concept is central to the TCM system and has since antiquity, been a guiding principle of both diagnosis and treatment. The 12 regular channels include: the 3 yin channels of the hand (lung, pericardium & heart), the 3 yang channels of the hand (large intestine, sanjiao, & small intestine), the 3 yang channels of the foot (stomach, gallbladder & urinary bladder), and the 3 yin channels of the foot (spleen, liver & kidney).

Please note that the anatomical "organ" name given to each channel does not represent the strict western concept of an anatomical structure, but more so, the philosophical and functional nature of specific and related tissues, vital substances, senses and emotions. At its core, TCM theory represents a *"landscape of functional relationships"* which provides integration of the human experience. Of the extra channels, our discussion will be limited to the Du, which is known as the *"sea of yang,"* and the Ren, which is known as the *"sea of yin."* These two extra channels thus represent the *confluence* or joining of all the yang or yin channels. According to TCM theory, Chi flows through each of the 12 regular channels in a fixed order, supplying both internal and external structures. *(see the previous chart for channel/organ times)* The Du and Ren channels function to regulate Chi within the yang and yin channels respectively. The channel system therefore, serves the physiological function of maintaining a harmonious coordination between the interior & exterior, and upper & lower portions of the body. Additionally, the channels serve to transport Chi & blood, nourish, and defend against exogenous pathogenic factors.

Points *(tsubo)* are specific sites through which the Chi of the Yin and Yang organs and channels is transported to the surface of the body. They are also described as the specific locations where Chi enters, leaves, joins, or converges. The literal translation of the Chinese character for "acupoint" *(shu-xue)* means "transportation hole." The 365 points of the body have empirically been assigned to a particular channel, which in turn is associated with a specific organ. Nearly five thousand years of observation has established both the location and action of each point. Clinically, the points are therefore locations where needles, pressure, massage (tui na), scraping (gua sha), suction (cupping), herbs, or moxa are applied to treat disease. Local and remote (distant) therapeutic properties are a basic feature of points found on the 12 regular channels. Painful or tender points and areas, which have no fixed specific location, are called "ashi" points. Anatomical landmarks are commonly used to define the location of fixed points. A system for measurement that accounts for individual differences has been devised. This system divides body parts into increments called "cun." A cun is equal to the distance between the two medial creases of the interphalangeal joint of the receiver's middle finger. An alternate method states that the width of the interphalangeal joint of the receiver's thumb is equal to 1-cun. The width of the receiver's four fingers when held together, at the level of the dorsal skin crease of the proximal interphalangeal joint of the middle finger, is considered to be equal to 3-cun. The distance between the transverse carpal crease and the transverse cubital crease is considered to be 12-cun. By using anatomical landmarks, known points, dividing or multiplying fixed distances, and palpation, a practitioner can quickly locate most points.

Necessary for an understanding of TCM anatomy and physiology is also the concept of the "Vital Substances." The vital substances not only include the bioenergy force Chi, including *original chi, food chi* or *Gu chi, gathering chi* or *Zong chi, true chi* or *Zhen chi, nutritive chi* or *Ying chi, defensive chi* or *Wei chi,* and *central chi* or *Zhong chi,* but also (the more physical) Blood, Essence *(Jing),* often associated with kidney and various thin and thick body fluids. Blood in TCM, is itself a more dense and material form of Chi derived from food and air. The primary function of Blood is to nourish. Essence or Jing is a precious substance, which is gained in limited amounts from one's parents, from food, drink, and the air one breathes. Essence is primarily stored in the kidneys. It forms the basis of growth, development, and reproduction. As Essence declines (with aging or use), so do one's stamina, sexual energy, and fertility. The thin, clear, and light *(jin)* body fluids are primarily used to moisten & nourish the skin and muscles. These thin fluids also manifest as tears, saliva, and mucous. The more thick, turbid, dense, and heavy *(ye)* body fluids are primarily used to moisten the joints, spine, brain, and bone marrow. These thick fluids also serve to lubricate the eyes, ears, nose, and mouth.

C. TCM Pathology, Assessment, & Diagnosis

TCM pathology is based upon acquired imbalances within the various channels and their associated tissues of Chi, Essence, blood, or other body fluids. The correct direction of movement of the various types of Chi or other substances depend upon the internal organs and any disruption in the flow of these must therefore, be viewed as a dysfunction of those organs. Clinically, disease processes of internal organs may also be reflected superficially to their corresponding body surfaces.

Etiological factors are usually described in TCM as being external, internal, or other. External causes of disease are due to climatic factors and have much to do with weather and seasonal changes. When protective or defensive *(Wei)* Chi *(of the Lung)* is weak, exogenous (external) pathogenic factors *(wind, cold, heat, damp, dryness)* may invade the body. When this type of invasion occurs, the channels may become pathways for transmitting disease from the superficial portion of the body to the interior. Internal causes of disease include constitutional factors such as the parent's health at conception, pre-natal influences, childhood conditions, and experiences (diet, trauma, exposure, etc.). As an adult, the internal cause of disease is considered to be the prolonged and intense experiencing of emotions including anger, joy, worry, pensiveness, sadness, fear, and shock. Each emotion has a particular effect on Chi and affects a specific channel or organ.

The "other" causes of disease are considered to be a weak constitution, fatigue/overexertion, excess sexual activity, improper diet, trauma, parasites or poisons, and receiving the wrong *(iatragenic)* treatment.

TCM diagnosis is accomplished through a sophisticated system of examination. The examination includes four methods described as Looking, Hearing (& smelling), Asking, and Feeling. Correct diagnosis is based upon a complex whole-person assessment using all of the four methods of examination. Patterns of disease are identified and categorized according to a number of parameters. These parameters include the: *(1)* Chi, Blood & Body Fluids, *(2)* Internal Organs, *(3)* Channels, *(4)* Pathogenic factors, *(5)* Five Elements, *(6)* Six Stages, (7) Four Levels, *(8)* Three Burners and *(9)* Eight Principles. Identification of disease via the Eight Principles involves using the categories of Yin/Yang, Hot/Cold, Excess/Deficient, and Interior/Exterior.

Treatment considerations with any TCM modality must take into account the correct TCM diagnosis, which necessitates a clinical assessment made using one or all the above described methods.

D. 14 Channels & Points

The following illustrations depict the twelve regular channels, two extra channels *(Du & Ren)* and their associated points. Of special interest are the beginning and ending points of each meridian. It is important to note the location of the channel in relation to the (western) anatomical structures it traverses.

LUNG CHANNEL

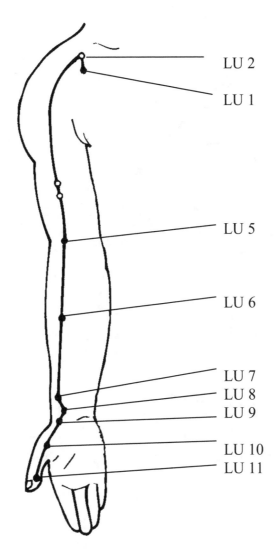

LU 2

LU 1

LU 5

LU 6

LU 7
LU 8
LU 9

LU 10
LU 11

LUNG CHANNEL

Common nomenclature: LU   *(Yin, Metal, 3am - 5am)*
Location: The Lung channel emerges, on lateral aspect of chest, 6-cun lateral to midline
and 1-cun below the hollow of the delto-pectoral triangle at LU-1. The channel ascends
one rib space to LU-2 and descends down the anterio-lateral aspect of the upper arm to
the cubital crease of the elbow, lateral to the bicep brachii tendon (LU-5). It continues to
descend along the radial artery to the wrist (LU-9), transverses the thenar mound and
terminates at the radial side of the thumbnail (LU-11). The Lung channel functions to
"govern Qi" and respiration, control the skin, regulate water passage (body fluids), and to
house the Corporeal Soul. The Lungs open into the nose. The Lungs are the most exterior
of the organs and are most sensitive to external pathogenic influences such as Wind,
Heat, Fire, Cold, Dampness and Dryness. Lung channel points are commonly used to
treat respiratory conditions, insomnia, weakness, night & day sweats, fever, headache,
body aches, and complexion problems.

LARGE INTESTINE CHANNEL

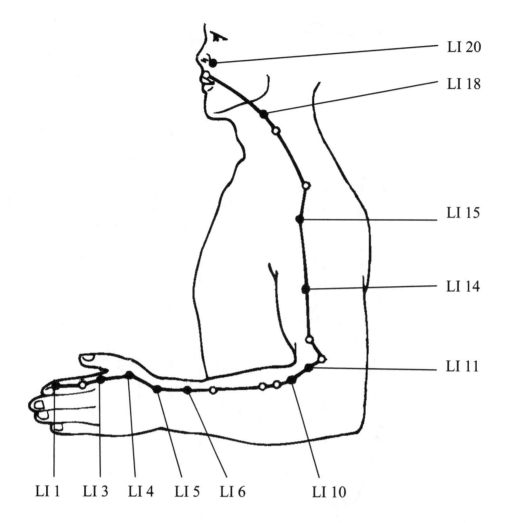

LI 20
LI 18
LI 15
LI 14
LI 11

LI 1   LI 3   LI 4   LI 5   LI 6   LI 10

LARGE INTESTINE CHANNEL

Common nomenclature: LI   *(Yang, Metal, 5am -7am)*
Location: The Large Intestine channel begins at the radial side of the tip of the index
finger (LI-1). It runs along this finger and passes through the interspace between the 1st
and 2nd metacarpal bones (LI-4) until it reaches the anatomical snuffbox at the depression
between the tendons of extensor pollicis longus and Brevis (LI-5). It ascends the lateral
aspect of the arm to the shoulder joint and into the depression between the scapular spine
and the lateral extremity of the clavicle (LI-16). The channel travels medially along the
lateral aspect of the neck and ascends to the cheek and passes underneath of the nose. It
terminates on the opposite side of the body at the naso-labial groove (LI-20). The Large
Intestine functions to receive food and drink from the Small Intestine & to excrete waste
food materials. The Large Intestine is quite sensitive to the pathogenic influences of Cold
& Damp. Large Intestine points are commonly used to treat digestive system problems,
vomiting, urinary disorders, fever, and abdominal pain.

STOMACH CHANNEL

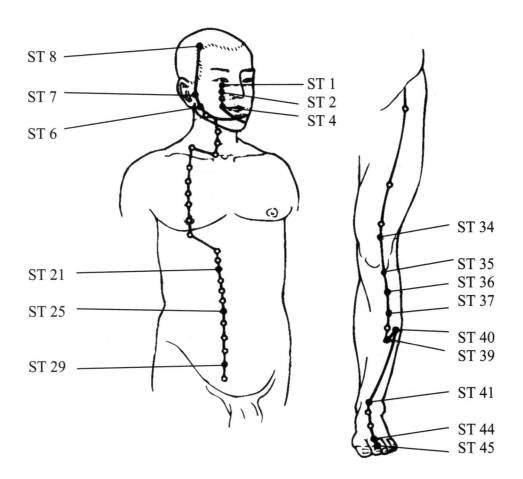

ST 8
ST 7
ST 6

ST 1
ST 2
ST 4

ST 21
ST 25
ST 29

ST 34
ST 35
ST 36
ST 37
ST 40
ST 39
ST 41
ST 44
ST 45

STOMACH CHANNEL

Common nomenclature: ST   *(Yang, Earth, 7am – 9am)*
Location: The Stomach channel begins at the infra-orbital ridge of the eye (ST-1) and descends down the cheek, runs under the nose, and back out to the corner of the mouth (ST-4). It continues along the jaw ascending in front of the ear to the upper corner of the hairline (ST-8). The channel descends internally and emerges along the anterior border of the sternocleidomastoid muscle (ST-9) to the superior border of the clavicle and moves to 4 cun lateral of the midline, on the mammillary line. It continues the descent below the breasts and moves inferior to 2-cun lateral to the midline until it reaches the inguinal region (ST-30). It descends along the lateral aspect of the femur to a point inferior & lateral to the patella (ST-35) and down the lateral side of the tibia (ST-36). The channel progresses inferiorly to the apex of the dorsum of the foot (ST-43) to terminate on the medial side of the 2nd toe (ST-45). The Stomach functions to transform & transport food and to assist in the descending of Qi. It is the origin of all the bodily fluids. The Stomach is sensitive to the pathogenic influences of Cold and Dryness, poor dietary habits, and conditions of excess & deficiency. Stomach channel points are commonly used to treat weakness, mouth & digestive system problems, and anorexia.

SPLEEN CHANNEL

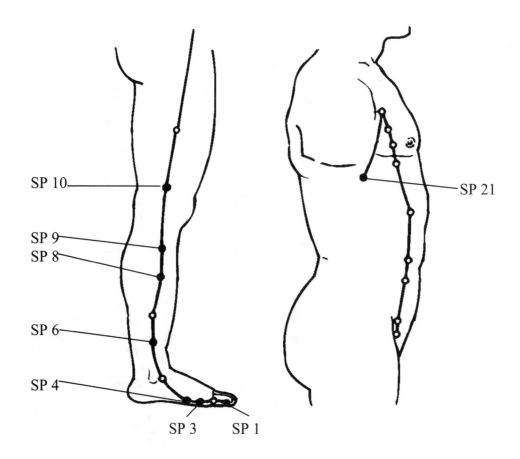

SP 10

SP 9

SP 8

SP 6

SP 4

SP 3   SP 1

SP 21

SPLEEN CHANNEL

Common nomenclature: SP   *(Yin, Earth, 9am – 11am)*
Location: The Spleen channel begins at the medial side of the tip of the big toe (SP-1)
and runs along the medial aspect of the foot, following the border where the skin changes
color. It ascends in front of the medial malleoulus and follows the posterior border of the
tibia up the medial aspect of the leg. It ascends up the abdomen and zigzags across it
several times moving laterally from 4-cun to 6-cun from the midline. It terminates at the
7th intercostals space on the mid-axillary line (SP-21). The main function of the Spleen is
to assist the Stomach in the process of digestion (transportation and transformation).
The Spleen is the primary organ involved in production of Chi. It controls the blood, the
muscles, and the four limbs. The spleen opens into the mouth and manifests in the lips. It
houses the mind. The Spleen is easily vexed by external dampness and cold from climatic
exposure or dietary indiscretion. Prolonged mental strain and brooding can weaken the
Spleen. Spleen related disorders include digestive complaints, anorexia, lassitude,
chilliness, edema, prolapse of internal organs, headache, dizziness, menstrual
dysfunction, low-grade fever, spontaneous sweating, scanty urine, bleeding, and anemia.
Spleens points alone or in combination with those of ST, BL, Ren, LI or LU are
commonly used to treat Spleen related disorders.

HEART CHANNEL

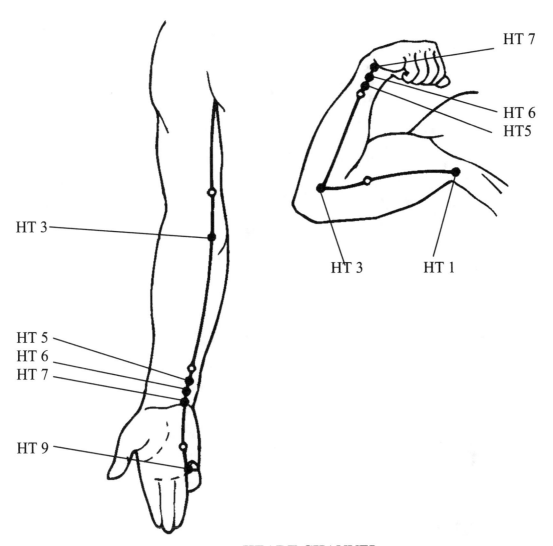

HEART CHANNEL

Common nomenclature: HT *(Yin, Fire, 11am – 1pm)*
Location: The heart channel emerges in the axilla (HT-1) and descends along the anterior medial aspect of the arm to the pisiform bone of the wrist (HT-7). It travels through the palm to the radial side of the little finger and terminates at the radial corner of the nail (HT-9). The Heart is known as the ruler of all the internal organs, functioning to govern the blood and blood vessels. The heart houses the mind (Shen) and also controls the sweat. The heart opens into the tongue and manifests in the complexion. The Heart is the least sensitive to external influences, yet is quite vulnerable to the emotional aspects of excess joy, sadness, and anger (frustration, resentment & depression). Heart channel points are used to treat; coma, palpitations, shortness of breath, angina, cyanosis, inappropriate sweating, tiredness, anemia, coldness of extremities, insomnia, vertigo, dream disturbed sleep, poor memory, anxiety, depression, and oral ulcers.

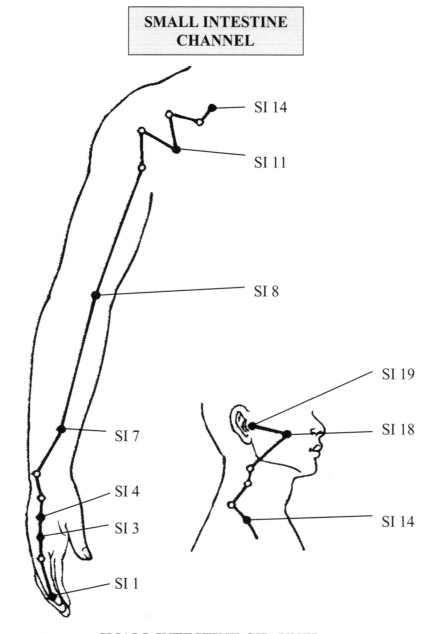

SMALL INTESTINE CHANNEL

Common nomenclature: SI *(Yang, Fire, 1pm – 3-pm)*
Location: The Small Intestine channel originates at the ulnar side of the tip of the little finger at the ulnar border of the nail (SI-1) and ascends along the ulnar aspect of the hand to reach the wrist at the styloid process of the ulna. It follows the anterior border of the ulna to the epicondyle of the Humerus (SI-8). The channel ascends the posterior aspect of the upper arm to the posterior joint of the shoulder. It zigzags across the scapula moving medially toward the spine. It then reverses direction and crosses the neck and cheek and terminates in the depression between the middle of the tragus of the ear and the condyloid process of the mandible (SI-19). The Small Intestine channel functions to control receiving and transforming of food from the stomach and to separate fluids. The Small Intestine channel is sensitive to dietary habits and emotional problems. Small Intestine points are commonly used in the treatment abdominal & urinary complaints.

BLADDER CHANNEL

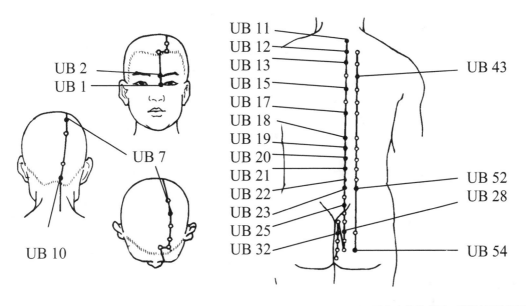

UB 11
UB 12
UB 13
UB 15
UB 17
UB 18
UB 19
UB 20
UB 21
UB 22
UB 23
UB 25
UB 32

UB 2
UB 1
UB 7
UB 10

UB 43
UB 52
UB 28
UB 54

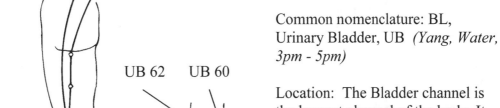

UB 62   UB 60
UB 39
UB 40
UB 57
UB 58
UB 60
UB 67   UB 65

BLADDER CHANNEL

Common nomenclature: BL, Urinary Bladder, UB *(Yang, Water, 3pm - 5pm)*

Location: The Bladder channel is the longest channel of the body. It begins at the inner canthus of the eye and ascends along the forehead to the vertex of the head running 2-cun lateral to the midline. It descends the back running 1.5-cun lateral the midline until it reaches the sacrum. It continues descending down the buttock to the popliteal crease (BL-40).

There is a 2nd branch of the Bladder meridian that descends the back at 3-cun lateral to the midline (BL-41) and enters the sacral foreman. It descends the leg and meets up with the 1st branch at the popliteal crease. The channel continues down the center of the calf, moving to the posterior lateral malleoulus (BL-60). It follows the 5th metatarsal bone and terminates at the lateral side of the tip of the 5th toe at the lateral border of the nail (BL-67). The functions of the Bladder include those of Chi transformation, i.e. the transforming and excreting of fluids. The Bladder is sensitive to cold and damp weather and to the effects of fear. Excessive sexual activity or unspoken feelings of suspicion and jealousy can harm the Bladder leading to urinary disorders, low back pain, lethargy, and a rapid pulse. Bladder points are often used in conjunction with those of the Spleen, Du, and Ren in treating the above-described conditions.

KIDNEY CHANNEL

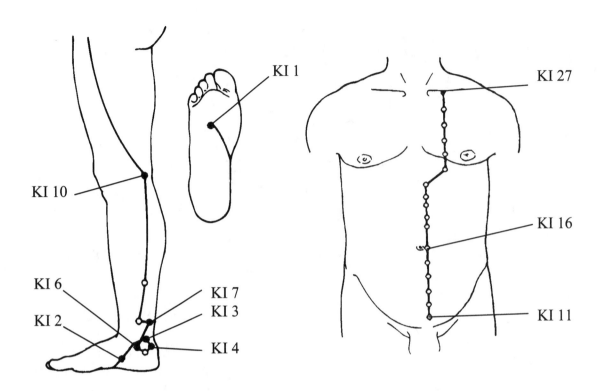

KI 1

KI 27

KI 10

KI 16

KI 6

KI 7

KI 3

KI 2

KI 4

KI 11

KIDNEY CHANNEL

Common nomenclature: KI   *(Yin, Water, 5pm - 7pm)*
Location: The Kidney channel begins on the sole of the foot between the 2nd and 3rd metatarsal bones, one third of the distance between the base of the 2nd toe and the heel (KI-1). It crosses the sole and runs anterior and inferior to the navicular tuberosity and travels posterior to the medial malleoulus (KI-3). It zigzags below the malleoulus and begins its ascent along the medial aspect of the leg to the popliteal crease. It ascends the abdomen from 5-cun below the umbilicus (KI-11) to 6-cun above the umbilicus (KI_21) and is 0.5-cun lateral to the midline. At the 5th intercostals space, the path moves to 2-cun lateral to the midline and terminates at the lower border of the clavicle (KI-27). The Kidney is referred to as the *Root of Life* and functions to primarily store "essence" and to govern birth, growth & reproduction. Secondarily the Kidney functions to control the bones, nourish the brain, govern water, and to receive Chi from the Lungs. TCM theory states that the Kidney cannot have an excess condition, but only those of deficiency. The Kidneys open into the ears, and thus exert influence on them. The Kidneys also influence the growth and health of the hair. The Kidneys are sensitive to hereditary weaknesses, fear, excess sexual activity, overwork, and aging. Kidney points are used to treat conditions of back pain, sexual dysfunction, urinary disorders, edema of the lower extremities, lassitude, and anorexia. Tinnitus, vertigo, osteoporosis, graying of the hair, and some respiratory disorders might also involve Kidney related conditions.

PERICARDIUM CHANNEL

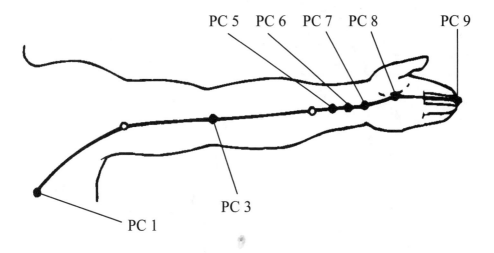

PC 5   PC 6   PC 7   PC 8   PC 9

PC 3

PC 1

PERICARDIUM CHANNEL

Common nomenclature: PC, Heart Protector, Heart Warmer, HP *(Yin, Fire, 7pm – 9pm)*
Location: The Pericardium channel begins on the chest, 1-cun lateral and slightly
superior to the nipple, in the 4th intercostals space (PC-1). It arches over the axilla and
travels along the anterio-medial aspect of the forearm. The channel continues descending
between the tendons of the palmaris longus and the flexor carpi radialis muscles (PC-6).
It crosses the palm to terminate at the tip of the middle finger (PC-9). The pericardium is
closely related to the heart. It functions to protect the heart from external pathogenic
factors. In terms of therapy, the Pericardium has more influence on the Heart than any
other channel. The Pericardium's influence is especially powerful with regard to
disorders of the chest cavity and emotional distress related to interpersonal relationships.
Pericardium points are commonly used to treat sun/heat stroke, angina, palpitation &
arrhythmias, seizures, nausea & vomiting (morning sickness or motion sickness),
uterine/menstrual disorders, severe anxiety, depression, bipolar disorder, aphasia, high
fevers, dry mouth, and tongue ulcers.

SAN JIAO CHANNEL (TRIPLE BURNER)

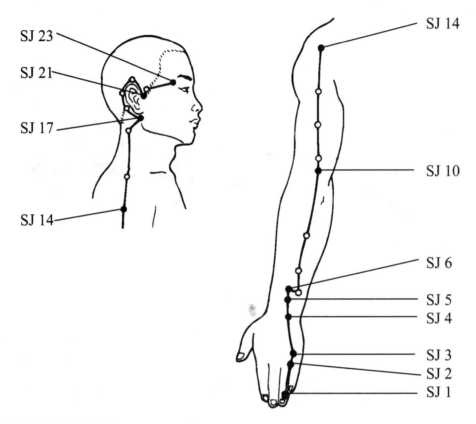

SJ 23
SJ 21
SJ 17
SJ 14

SJ 14
SJ 10
SJ 6
SJ 5
SJ 4
SJ 3
SJ 2
SJ 1

SAN JIAO CHANNEL

Common nomenclature: SJ, Triple Warmer, TW, Triple Heater, TH
(Yang, Fire, 9pm - 11pm)
Location: The San Jiao channel begins on the dorsal aspect of the ring finger at the ulnar border of the nail (SJ-1). It runs between the 4th and 5th metacarpal bones along the posterior of the hand and ascends the forearm between the radius and the ulna. It crosses the olecranon and ascends the posterior aspect of the upper arm to the origin of the deltoid muscle (SJ-14). The channel moves medially along the trapezius muscle and ascends the neck on the posterior border of the Sternocleidomastoid muscle (SJ-16). It travels behind the earlobe (SJ-17) and circles the border of the ear just inside the hairline. It continues to a point 0.5-cun anterior to the upper border of the root of the ear (SJ-22) and terminates in the depression on the supraorbital margin, at the lateral end of the eyebrow. San Jiao is composed of the Upper, Middle, and Lower Burners (Jiao) which, are compared to a "mist," a "bubbling cauldron," and a "drainage ditch" respectively. San Jiao functions to receive and transport fluids and nourishment, excrete wastes, and control the distribution of the various types of Chi. San Jiao points are commonly used to treat depression, irritability & mood swings, fever & chills, sore throat, ear aches, deafness, tinnitus, blurred vision, headaches, herpes *(Zoster & Simplex),* Bell's Palsy, local pain & stiffness of the head, neck, shoulder, and arm.

GALL BLADDER CHANNEL

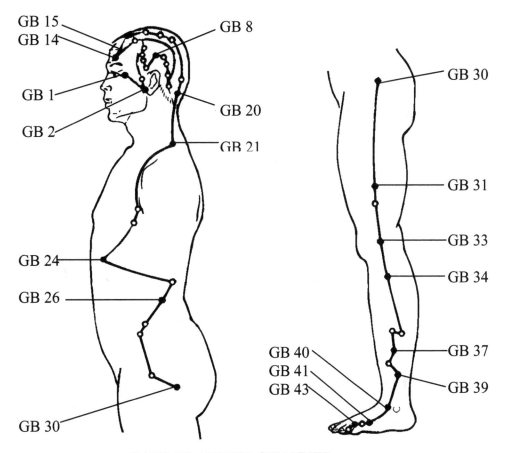

GB 15
GB 14
GB 8
GB 1
GB 20
GB 2
GB 21
GB 30
GB 31
GB 33
GB 34
GB 24
GB 26
GB 40
GB 37
GB 41
GB 43
GB 39
GB 30

GALL BLADDER CHANNEL

Common nomenclature: GB *(Yang, Wood, 11pm – 1am)*
Location: The Gall Bladder channel originates 0.5-cun lateral to the outer cantus of the eye (GB-1). It moves laterally to the intertragic notch ascending within the hairline and zigzagging the head while circling along the posterior margin of the ear. The channel descends into the abdomen from the occiput (GB-20) and runs along the trapezius muscle (GB-21) and down the mid-axillary line. It zigzags on the abdomen to the tip of the 12th rib (GB-25) and then to the tip of the 11th rib (GB-26). It remains lateral to the hip joint and descends along the lateral aspect of the thigh to the tender depression 1 cun anterior and inferior to the head of the fibula (GB-34). It continues its descent to the lateral malleolus following the dorsal surface of the foot along the groove between the 4th and 5th metatarsals. The channel terminates at the lateral side of the 4th toe at the base of the nail (GB-44). The Gall Bladder functions to receive store and excrete bile. This function is described as being an expression of the Liver's role of ensuring the smooth flow of Chi and is especially important to the healthy functioning of the sinews. The Gall Bladder also functions to impart courage and control one's ability to make decisions. Points are used to treat headaches, tinnitus, vertigo, deafness, eye problems, speech disorders, insomnia, Bell's Palsy, Sciatica, and particularly ligament, tendon, and muscle disorders.

LIVER CHANNEL

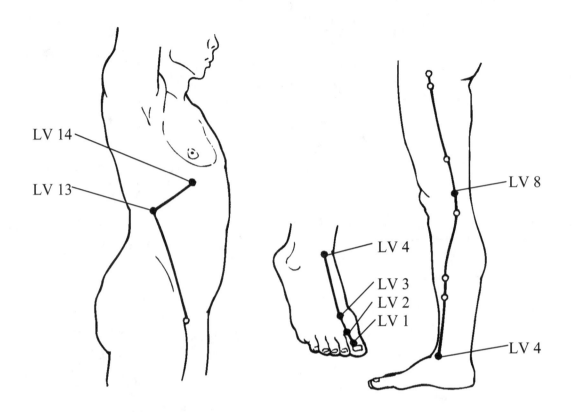

LIVER CHANNEL

Common nomenclature: LV (*Yin, Wood, 1am – 3am*)
Location: The Liver channel on the dorsal aspect of the big toe on the lateral side of the corner of the nail (LV-1). It travels between the 1st and 2nd metatarsal bones to the anterior border of the medial malleolus. It ascends the medial aspect of the calf along the posterior border of the tibia to a point just superior to the medial end of the popliteal crease (LV-8). The channel ascends the thigh to the crease of the groin, medial to the femoral vein (LV-12). It terminals on the mammillary line, in the 6th intercostal space, 4-cun lateral to the midline (LV-14). The Liver channel stores blood, ensures the smooth movement of Chi and controls the sinews. It opens into the eyes and manifests in the nails. The Liver houses the "Ethereal Soul." The Liver is vulnerable to the external pathogenic factors of Wind & Dampness, excess emotions of anger, resentment & irritation, and dietary indiscretions. Liver points are commonly used in treating mood disorders, hypertension, aphasia, headache, nausea, vertigo, tinnitus & deafness, eye disorders, digestive complaints, menstrual & genital disorders, fever, stroke, tremors, convulsions & meningitis, and muscular atrophy, weakness or cramping.

DU CHANNEL
(GOVERNING VESSEL)

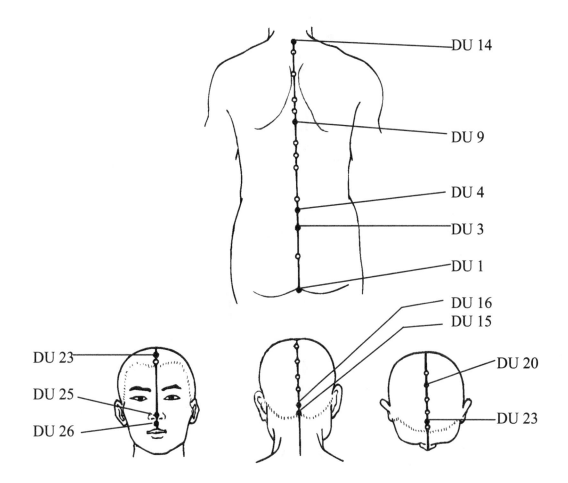

DU CHANNEL

Common nomenclature: Du, Governing Vessel, GV   *(Yang)*
Location: The Du channel (meridian) begins on the midline of the body, midway
between the tip of the coccyx and the anus (DU-1). It travels posterior along the midline
of the sacrum and the interior spinal column to the nape of the neck (DU-14). It ascends
to the vertex of the head (DU-20) and begins its descend along the midline to the bridge
of the nose and philtrum (DU-26). It terminates inside of the mouth, in the superior
frenulum, at the junction of the upper lip and the gum (DU-28). The Du channel is called
the "Sea of Yang" and thus, exerts an influence on all the Yang channels & organs. The
Du channel also functions to nourish the spine & brain. Points of the Du channel might
be used to treat conditions such as vertigo, tinnitus, low back pain, poor memory,
seizures, stiff neck, and fever.

REN CHANNEL
(CONCEPTION VESSEL)

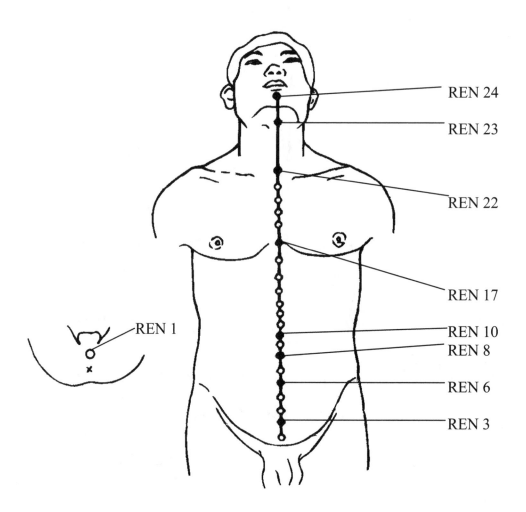

REN 24

REN 23

REN 22

REN 17

REN 10

REN 8

REN 6

REN 3

REN 1

REN CHANNEL

Common nomenclature: Ren, Conception Vessel, CV *(Yin)*
Location: The Ren channel (meridian) begins at the perineum, midway between the anus and scrotum in men and the anus and the posterior labial commissure in women (REN-1). It ascends the midline of the abdomen from the superior border of the pubic symphysis to the suprasternal notch (REN-22). It continues up the midline of the neck and terminates in the center of the mentolabial groove above the chin (REN-24). The Ren channel is called the "Sea of Yin" and is the confluence (joining) of all the Yin channels. The Ren channel functions to exert an influence on all the Yin channels of the body. It is of great importance for regulation of the reproductive systems of both men and women. Ren channel points are typically used in treating conditions of fertility, pregnancy, childbirth, menstruation, menopause, tumors, hernias, asthma, and other conditions of the abdomen, thorax, lungs, throat, and face.

Review Questions - Human Anatomy, Physiology & Kinesiology

1. A bladder infection spreads upwards to the kidneys through which structures?
   a) Ureters
   b) Glomerulus
   c) Urethra
   d) Pyloric Sphincter

2. Which muscle is associated with supination of the forearm?
   a) Coracobrachialis
   b) Triceps Brachii
   c) Biceps Brachii
   d) Brachioradialis

3. Slightly moveable joints connected by discs of cartilage are known as:
   a) Synarthrotic
   b) Diarthrotic
   c) Bursae
   d) Amphiarthrotic

4. Rhythmic waves of muscular contraction that occur in the walls of various tubular organs and help to propel food through the digestive system:
   a) Polarization
   b) Peristalsis
   c) Fibrillation
   d) Twitch

5. This joint permits biaxial movements and exists only between the carpal and metacarpal bones of the thumb:
   a) Ellipsoidal
   b) Saddle
   c) Gliding
   d) Hinge

6. The insertion of the sternocleidomastoid is the:
   a) Sternum
   b) Hyoid
   c) Clavicle
   d) Mastoid Process

7. The most superficial abdominal muscle on the anterior surface of the body is the:
   a) Rectus Abdominis
   b) Transverse Abdominis
   c) Internal Oblique
   d) External Oblique

8. The most abundant tissue in the body is:
   a) Epithelial
   b) Muscular
   c) Connective
   d) Nervous

9. Quadrant of the abdomen in which the liver is located:
   a) Upper Left
   b) Lower Right
   c) lower Left
   d) Upper Right

10. The action of the teres minor is:
    a) Medial rotation of humerus
    b) Lateral rotation of humerus
    c) Flexion of humerus
    d) Flexion of forearm

11. A substance such as a blood clot or bubble of gas that is carried by the blood and obstructs a blood vessel is known as a(n):
    a) Arteriosclerosis
    b) Infarct
    c) Phlebitis
    d) Embolus

12. A cord or sheet of connective tissue by which two or more bones are bound together at a joint:
    a) Linea Alba
    b) Tendon
    c) Ligament
    d) Aponeurosis

13. Which is not a function of the liver?
    a) End digestion of proteins
    b) Produces bile
    c) Storage of vitamins
    d) Removal of toxic substances from body fluids

14. Necrosis of heart muscle from ischemia is known as a "heart attack"or:
    a) Angina Pectoris
    b) Coronary Bypass
    c) Myocardial Infarction
    d) Aneurysm

15. Valve located between the left atrium and left ventricle which is sometimes damaged from rheumatic fever:
    a) Aortic Semilunar
    b) Pulmonary Semilunar
    c) Tricuspid
    d) Bicuspid (Mitral)

16. An excessive accumulation of fluid within the interstitial space is known as:
    a) Plasma
    b) Interstitial Serum
    c) Lymph
    d) Edema

17. Descending order of the small intestine:
    a) Fundus, Duodenum, Jejunum
    b) Jejunum, Ileum, Duodenum
    c) Duodenum, Jejunum, Ileum
    d) Pyloris, Jejunum, Ileum

18. Phase of the cardiac cycle during which a heart chamber wall is relaxed:
    a) Hyperbole
    b) Systole
    c) Cardiac Atony
    d) Diastole

19. Endocrine glands located on the top of the kidneys:
    a) Adrenal
    b) Pineal
    c) Pancreas
    d) Parathyroid

20. Part of the brain responsible for muscular coordination and balance:
    a) Brain Stem
    b) Cerebellum
    c) Diencephalon
    d) Cerebrum

21. Mineral required to facilitate the attraction of actin and myosin within a muscle fiber:
    a) Sodium
    b) Phosphorus
    c) Magnesium
    d) Calcium

22. Artery located behind the knee supplying blood to the knee joint and certain muscles in the thigh and calf:
    a) Femoral
    b) Popliteal
    c) Posterior Tibial
    d) Internal Iliac

23. Nerve bundle, which passes between the anterior and middle scalene muscles as it moves toward the axilla:
    a) Cervical Plexus
    b) Lumbosacral Plexus
    c) Brachial Plexus
    d) Phrenic Nerves

24. Hypertonicity of this muscle can put undue pressure on the sciatic nerve bundle resulting in pain or numbness radiating down the posterior thigh and leg:
    a) Gluteus Maximus
    b) Tensor Fascia Lata
    c) Iliopsoas
    d) Piriformis

25. Medial and lateral bony projections located at the distal end of the tibia and fibula:
    a) Malleoli
    b) Condyle
    c) Patella
    d) Tubercle

26. The longest vein in the body originating on the medial aspect of the foot and extending upward along the medial side of the leg toward the inguinal ligament:
    a) Popliteal
    b) Femoral
    c) Great Saphenous
    d) Anterior Tibial

27. The most superficial layer of meninges composed primarily of tough, white fibrous connective tissue:
    a) Pia Mater
    b) Arachnoid Mater
    c) Dura Mater
    d) Cerebrospinal Layer

28. Avascular tissue with very little intercellular matrix specializing in absorption, secretion, and protection:
    a) Nervous
    b) Epithelial
    c) Connective
    d) Areolar

29. Transports deoxygenated blood from the right ventricle into the lungs for oxygenation:
    a) Pulmonary Arteries
    b) Right Coronary Arteries
    c) Right Coronary Veins
    d) Pulmonary Veins

30. Muscular contraction in which the muscle shortens:
    a) Isotonic
    b) Tetanic
    c) Antagonist
    d) Isometric

31. Which muscle is located on the posterior surface of the lower leg, crossing two joints and is responsible for plantar flexion of the ankle?
    a) Rectus Femoris
    b) Soleus
    c) Gastrocnemius
    d) Popliteus

32. Serous membrane covering the surface of organs found in the body cavities:
    a) Parietal
    b) Mucous
    c) Synovial
    d) Visceral

33. Lymph collected from the majority of the body is routed to the left subclavian vein and ultimately the vena cava by this structure:
    a) Aorta
    b) Thoracic Duct
    c) Hepatic Portal Vein
    d) Pulmonary Vein

34. A diabetic patient who has unknowingly given himself too much insulin would likely be trying to balance their system by eating foods which contain:
    a) Protein
    b) Fat
    c) Potassium
    d) Glucose

35. The origin of the femoral nerve is:
    a) Lumbosacral Plexus
    b) Brachial Plexus
    c) Sciatic Notch
    d) Posterior Superior Iliac Spine

36. This muscle is responsible for stabilizing the scapula against the chest wall:
    a) Pectoralis Major
    b) Pectoralis Minor
    c) Subscapularis
    d) Serratus Anterior

37. This vessel arises from the aorta and delivers oxygenated blood to the myocardium:
    a) Pulmonary Arteries
    b) Pulmonary Veins
    c) Coronary Arteries
    d) Coronary Veins

38. The pyloric valve is located between:
    a) Aorta/ventricle
    b) Esophagus/stomach
    c) Small/large intestines
    d) Stomach/small intestine

39. Stimulation of the parasympathetic nervous system causes:
    a) Increased heart rate
    b) Decreased heart rate
    c) Death
    d) None of the above

40. Transmits nerve impulses from the brain to muscle:
    a) Sensory
    b) Arachnoid
    c) Motor
    d) Cecum

41. Vitamin "D" is synthesized in the:
    a) Skin
    b) Muscle tissue
    c) Bone
    d) Hair

42.   Increasing the angle of a joint is:
        a) Flexion
        b) Rotations
        c) Circumduction
        d) Extension

43.   Non-movable type of joint is:
        a) Diarthrosis
        b) Synarthrosis
        c) Amphiarthrosis
        d) None of the above

44.   Part of the brain controlling the "Vital Functions":
        a) Cerebrum
        b) Diencephalon
        c) Cerebellum
        d) Brain stem

45.   The functional unit of the kidney for urine production:
        a) Adrenal
        b) Nephron
        c) Ureter
        d) Urethra

46.   Which of the following muscles acts with the piriformis to externally rotate the
        femur?
        a) Gracilis
        b) Obturator externus
        c) Pectineus
        d) Psoas major

47.   Which is not normally reabsorbed by the kidney tubules?
        a) Water
        b) Glucose
        c) Urea
        d) Protein

48.   The circulation of blood from the right ventricle through the pulmonary artery to
        the lung is called:
        a) Renal circulation
        b) Portal circulation
        c) Systemic circulation
        d) Pulmonary circulation

49. Insulin is secreted by:
   a) Alpha cells
   b) Melanocytes
   c) Beta cells
   d) Sebaceous glands

50. Muscle contraction allowing for good posture is:
   a) Isotonic
   b) Isometric
   c) Tetanic
   d) Tonic

51. The cardiac sphincter is found at the distal end of the:
   a) Urethra
   b) Aorta
   c) Esophagus
   d) Motor neuron

52. Name of tissue found covering the articular surface of bones:
   a) Hyaline
   b) Pericardium
   c) Epidermis
   d) Periosteum

53. Also called the master gland:
   a) Thyroid
   b) Anterior pituitary
   c) Adrenal
   d) Pineal

54. Structure which initiates stretch reflex in muscle (causing contraction):
   a) Lysosome
   b) Spindle cell
   c) Precapillary sphincter
   d) None of the above

55. The three muscles that attach to the coracoid process are:
   a) Pectoralis major, pectoralis minor, and subclavius
   b) Pectoralis minor, long head of biceps, coracobrachialis
   c) Coracobrachialis, short head of biceps, pectoralis minor
   d) Coracobrachialis, short head of biceps, pectoralis major

56. During what kind of exercise does the tone of the muscle increase while its length remains the same?
    a) Isotonic
    b) Kinetic
    c) Isotopic
    d) Isometric

57. Where do the flexors of the wrist originate?
    a) Olecranon process
    b) Lateral process
    c) Medial epicondyle
    d) Radial tuberosity

58. Which of the following is a two joint muscle?
    a) Biceps brachii
    b) Brachialis
    c) Soleus
    d) Coracobrachialis

59. A lateral curve of the spine is a deviation known as:
    a) Lordosis
    b) Kyphosis
    c) Scoliosis
    d) Trichinosis

60. Inversion of the foot by the tibialis anterior turns the sole:
    a) Toward the midline
    b) Downward
    c) Away from the midline
    d) Upward

61. The rotator cuff is found at which joint in the body?
    a) Radioulnar joint
    b) Humeroulnar joint
    c) Sternoclavicular joint
    d) Scapulohumeral joint

62. Which type of muscle is responsible for movement of the bones?
    a) Involuntary
    b) Non-striated (smooth)
    c) Striated (skeletal)
    d) Branching (cardiac)

63. The only bone to bone attachment between the lower appendicular skeleton and the axial skeleton is the:
   a) Sternoclavicular joint
   b) Sacroiliac joint
   c) Glenohumeral joint
   d) Knee joint

64. The origin of the short head of the biceps brachii is:
   a) Coracoid process
   b) Ulnar tuberosity
   c) Radial tuberosity
   d) Supraglenoid tubercule

65. The most superficial muscle of the back is the:
   a) Trapezius
   b) Latissimus dorsi
   c) Rhomboids
   d) Erector spinae

66. The motion that can occur between the occiput and atlas is:
   a) Lateral rotation
   b) Lateral flexion
   c) Flexion and extension
   d) No motion

67. Brachialis is the strongest flexor of the:
   a) Wrist
   b) Humerus
   c) Hip
   d) Elbow

68. Which artery should you be aware of when working in the cervical area?
   a) Radial
   b) Femoral
   c) Carotid
   d) Brachial

69. The quadriceps muscle that attaches to the anterior inferior iliac spine is the:
   a) Vastus medialis
   b) Vastus lateralis
   c) Vastus intermedius
   d) Rectus femoris

70. The gluteal muscle that attaches to the iliotibial tract is the:
    a) Gluteus medius
    b) Gluteus maximus
    c) Gluteus minimus
    d) Gluteus intermedius

71. Which of the following muscles might need to be considered in assessment of the condition *Condromalacia Patella?*
    a) Tibialis anterior
    b) Tibialis posterior
    c) Rectus femoris
    d) Biceps femoris

72. Proprioceptor, which when stimulated by tension, causes a lengthening of its associated muscle:
    a) Muscle spindle cell
    b) Nociceptor
    c) St. John cell
    d) Golgi tendon organ

73. Which is an example of a "sesamoid" bone?
    a) Distal phalange of the 5th toe
    b) Patella
    c) Medial epicondyle
    d) Hyoid

74. Which type of cell plays a role in the body's defense against bacteria?
    a) Erythrocytes (RBC's)
    b) Thrombocytes (platelets)
    c) Leukocytes (WBC's)
    d) Fibrocytes (CT cells)

75. Which type of joint is the most mobile?
    a) Saddle
    b) Ball and socket
    c) Hinge
    d) Gliding

76. Which represents the normal amount of cervical rotation?
    a) 0 to 30 degrees
    b) 0 to 45 degrees
    c) 0 to 90 degrees
    d) 0 to 120 degrees

77. Name the organelle that is responsible for cellular energy production:
    a) Lysosome
    b) Golgi apparatus
    c) Mitochondria
    d) Smooth endoplasmic reticulum

78. Which point of muscle attachment is considered most movable?
    a) Proximal
    b) Origin
    c) Insertion
    d) None of the above

79. In TCM theory, which element is most associated with the Stomach Channel?
    a) Earth
    b) Metal
    c) Wood
    d) Wind

80. With your client supine on the table, where does the Stomach Channel run?
    a) Between Rectus Femoris and Vastus Medialis
    b) Between Semitendinosus & Vastus Medialis
    c) Between Rectus Femoris and Vastus Lateralis
    d) Between Rectus Femoris and Sartorius

81. When working on a client with upper back and cervical problems, you discover trigger points in the mid-upper Trapezius and at the Occipital Ridge, which TCM channel has points in these same areas?
    a) Liver
    b) Gall Bladder
    c) Stomach
    d) Spleen

82. In TCM theory, the anterior surface of the human body is considered to be more:
    a) Yin
    b) Yang
    c) Difficult to treat
    d) Appropriate location for treating males

83. Which of the following channels is considered to be the "confluence' of all the yang channels?
    a) Du (Governing vessel)
    b) Ren (Conception vessel)
    c) Stomach
    d) Large Intestine

84. Through which channel does Chi flow during the time period of 3am to 5am?
    a) Bladder
    b) Du
    c) Gall Bladder
    d) Lung

85. Which of the five elements is associated with the sound of "Laughing?"
    a) Wood
    b) Metal
    c) Fire
    d) Water

86. Which channel begins at a point on the radial side of the index finger, travels along the arm, the neck and face to end at a point on the opposite side of the body at the naso-labial groove?
    a) Stomach
    b) Spleen
    c) Kidney
    d) Large Intestine

87. Which is the longest channel of the body, is associated with the Water element, begins at the medial canthus of the eye, and ends at a point on the lateral side of the tip of the small toe?
    a) Kidney
    b) Bladder
    c) Liver
    d) Gall Bladder

88. Which channel begins at a point on the perineum, ascends the midline of the abdomen, and terminates at the mentolabial groove of the chin?
    a) Kidney
    b) Bladder
    c) Ren (Conception vessel)
    d) Du (Governing vessel)

89. With which organs (channels) is the element of Wood associated?
    a) Liver & Gall Bladder
    b) Stomach & Spleen
    c) Lung & large Intestine
    d) Heart & Small Intestine

90. With which organs (channels) is the season of summer associated?
    a) Liver & Gall Bladder
    b) Stomach & Spleen
    c) Lung & large Intestine
    d) Heart & Small Intestine

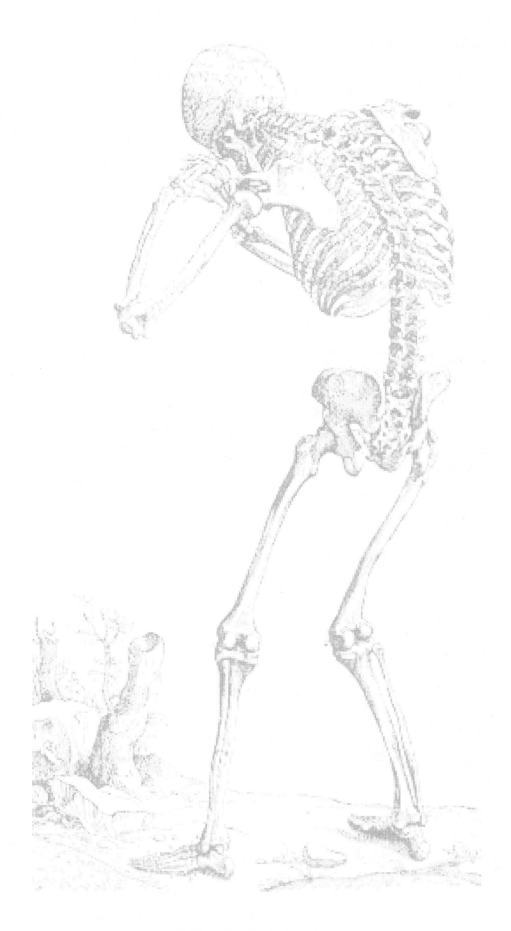

II. CLINICAL PATHOLOGY

A. Introduction to the Mechanisms of Disease and Healing

1. Terminology:

a. *Acute* - Disease or condition that appears suddenly and is usually of short duration.

b. *Chronic* - Disease or condition that develops slowly and lasts for a prolonged period of time (maybe for life).

c. *Diagnosis* - Name given to a patient's condition. Implies the illness will follow a prescribed course.

d. *Disease* - The abnormality in body function (lack of homeostasis). A morbid process which threatens the well-being of an organism.

e. *Endemic* - Disease that is natural to a local geographical region.

f. *Epidemic* - Disease occurring in many individuals in any region at the same time, widely diffused and spreading.

g. *Epidemiology* - Study of the occurrence, frequency, transmission, and distribution of a disease.

h. *Etiology* - The study of the origin (cause) of the disease.

i. *Health* - The state of optimal physical, mental, and emotional well being, not merely the absence of disease.

j. *Pandemic* - Epidemic effecting large geographic areas (global).

k. *Pathogenesis* - The pattern of a disease's development.

l. *Pathology* - The study of disease.

m. *Pathophysiology* - The study of the physiological process associated with disease.

n. *Prognosis* - The outcome of a disease (a prediction).

o. *Signs* - Objective abnormalities that can be observed by someone other than the patient.

p. *Symptoms* - Subjective abnormalities as reported by the patient.

q. *Syndrome* - A collection of signs and symptoms usually with a common etiology, which present a clear picture of a pathological condition.

2. Etiology of Disease:

a. *Trauma* - Damage caused by mechanical injury, chemical agents, extreme hot or cold, and radiation, which alter the normal homeostatic process.

b. *Infection* - Invasion of the body by pathogenic organisms such as virus, bacteria, fungus, and parasites. May cause disease by interfering with the normal functions of the host. Infectious agents may be spread by *Person-to-Person contact* (through air, direct contact - skin or body fluids, via contaminated materials), *Environmental contact* (food, water, soil, & assorted surfaces), *Opportunistic invasion* (pathogens are normal inhabitants of environment & waiting for an opportunity or advantage), or *Transmission by a vector* (another organism - tick, fly, mosquito).

c. *Degeneration* - Although a normal process of aging, overuse or trauma may facilitate an untimely breakdown of tissues.

d. *Neoplasm* - Abnormal tissue growth (tumor). May be *benign* - remain localized within the tissues from which they grow, surrounded by a capsule of dense tissue, and often grow slowly. Usually are not life threatening, but can be disruptive of normal function. May be *malignant* (cancerous) - tissue growth that can move to another part of the body and grow abnormally. Tissue growth of malignant tumors is generally more aggressive, usually not encapsulated, and tend to spread to other tissues. Tumor cells may migrate via either lymphatic or circulatory system in a process known as metastasis. Malignant tumors may also replace normal tissue in organs, thus causing great problems.

e. *Genetic/Congenital* - Abnormalities of development caused by faulty genetic program or due to noxious influences on the fetus in utero. Some congenital abnormalities are present a birth; others may appear later in life when stress of the environment causes symptoms to appear.

f. *Deficiency* - Disorders resulting from an imbalance of essential nutrients. Such disorders may be related to reduced nutrients in food sources or poor digestion and absorption.

g. *Auto-immunity* - Disorders resulting from an attack by the body's own immune system. The body makes a "mistake" in identifying one or more tissues as invading organisms and forms an antibody to that tissue. Closely related are deficiencies and hypersensitivity of the immune system.

h. Other than overt causes of disease we must consider that certain *predisposing conditions* make the onset of a disease process more likely. These **risk factors** may be categorized into several types:

> **1)** *Genetic Factors* - An inherited trait which puts a person at a greater risk of developing a specific disorder.
>
> **2)** *Lifestyle* - Work and living conditions may expose a group to higher risk. Sun exposure and dietary habits may lead to specific diseases.
>
> **3)** *Stress* - Physical and psychological challenges may lower one's immune response to disease, putting that person at greater risk. Nervous and endocrine system changes that result from stress may

predispose to a number of ailments. Chronic disease may dispose someone to additional ailments.

4) *Environment* - Factors such as air quality and climate influence the ability of our body to function normally and influence potential disease causing organisms with whom we share the environment.

5) *Age* - Physiological changes during the life cycle put humans at greater risk for developing certain disorders at certain times of their lives.

Risk factors often overlap, and having more than one risk factor present may increase the potential for developing a specific disease. Also note that many of the risk factors can be avoided, thus lowering the potential for developing a specific disease.

Diseases are further categorized as being either structural or functional. Structural disorders are characterized by structural changes within the body that represent the basic disease process. These disorders are known as organic diseases. The term lesion is used to describe a structural change and may be either micro or macroscopic.

Functional disorders are those that seemingly begin without the presence of any lesions. They are characterized by physiologic changes and subsequent symptoms. Insomnia due to anxiety illustrates this pathophysiological disease process.

3. Epidemiology: Frequency, Distribution, and Significance of Disease

Diseases are commonly discussed in terms of ***mortality*** and ***morbidity***. Mortality refers to the number of deaths caused by a particular disease, while morbidity refers to the frequency of the disability. Heart disease ranks number one as a killer of Americans followed closely by cancer. Stroke is the third leading cause of death in the U.S. followed by accidents and pulmonary disease.

Acute diseases are those that last for a short time (usually a few days to a few weeks). More than 50% of acute diseases are respiratory in nature. Of these, most are viral in origin. Injuries account for nearly a third of acute ailments. The frequency of acute illnesses appears to decrease with age.

Chronic diseases are conversely, those that have a long duration, often for a lifetime. The frequency of chronic disease dramatically increases with age. Chronic diseases are discussed in terms of prevalence, the proportion of a population, which has that condition at any one time. Periodontal disease and mental illness rank number one and two in terms of prevalence. The five most reported chronic diseases include arthritis, hearing impairment, hypertension, heart disease, and visual impairment. Note that all those previously mentioned ailments increase in frequency with age.

4. Injury, Inflammation, and Repair

Injury to a cell either results in recovery or *necrosis (*cell death). Reversible cell injury is characterized by preservation of the nucleus. Once the nucleus is destroyed or the cell membrane disrupted, the cell cannot recover. After cell death, enzymes contained in lysosomes digest the remaining cell structures. Cells can be injured by many causes. *Anoxia* (lack of oxygen) and *hypoxia* (reduced oxygen) represent the most common causes of cell necrosis. Chronic non-lethal cell injury may produce atrophy or other abnormal cellular changes.

Inflammation is the protective reaction produced by the body in response to cellular injury and necrosis. Vascular and cellular changes bring about the cardinal signs of inflammation including ***pain, heat, redness, swelling, and loss of function.*** The release of *histamine* from *mast* cells causes vasodilatation and increased permeability of small vessels, leading to a loss of fluid into surrounding tissue (*edema* - swelling). *Bradykinin* is formed and initiates a pain response. Increased blood flow (*hyperemia*) causes redness and heat. The effects of inflammation serve to destroy or limit the spread of an infective agent and to clean up damaged tissue in preparation for repair. White blood cells are chemically drawn to the area to assist in both defensive and clean-up duties (*chemotaxis*). Inflammation can be either acute or chronic. When the inflammatory response persists, a proliferation of new fibrous tissue occurs. Inflammatory conditions are often treated with non-steroidal (aspirin, ibuprofen, etc) or steroidal (cortisone, prednisone), anti-inflammatory drugs that block the synthesis of the inflammatory chemicals arachidonic acid and prostaglandin.

Tissue repair occurs through either ***regeneration or fibrosis.*** In *regeneration,* similar cells replace the destroyed tissue. Regeneration is the most desirable form of repair in that normal function is often restored. Tissues that are continuously replacing their cells have a greater capacity for regeneration. Epithelial and bone marrow tissue are examples. Most body tissues are slow to regenerate and some have no potential at all. Nervous and cardiac muscle cells cannot undergo cell division in adults and therefore, lack the ability to rebuild tissue. *Fibrosis* (scarring) can occur in any tissue, producing a tough, dense mass of collagen known as a scar. Repair by fibrosis does not restore normal function, but provides a strong bridge between the damaged area and normal tissue. The process of fibrosis (scarring) is carried on by *fibroblasts* which lay down collagen fibers which later contract, thus stabilizing the damaged area. When fibrous tissue proliferation does not stabilize the area, minerals are deposited into the tissue, forming calcium deposits or spurs.

B. Neoplasms and Hyperplasias - Proliferation of cells, with an increase in tissue mass.

1. Hyperplasia is an exaggerated response in cell growth to a stimulus, resulting in an *abnormal number* of cells. A non-exaggerated response to a stimulus, such as injury, is known as tissue repair. Hypertrophy means an increase in the size of cells, and is best applied to muscle tissue. Hyperplasia may result as a response to various stimuli such as inflammation, hormonal imbalances, or chronic irritation (swollen lymph nodes, thyroid goiter, and calluses are examples).

2. Neoplasms - (*neo,* new & *plasm,* matter) known as tumors, are growths that proliferate independently of normal cellular control mechanisms. They are presumed to arise from altered (mutated) genetic conditions and function as if they were independent parasitic organisms at odds with their host. Like hyperplasias, most neoplasms arise from cells that undergo physiologic replacement and may come from embryonic or somatic tissue cells. The ability of a cell to be replaced contributes to the likelihood of that tissue type to develop a neoplasm (epithelial cells undergo continuous replacement, cardiac muscle cells cannot be replaced). Most neoplasms contain only a single cell type (connective, epithelial, muscle, etc.), yet some tumors that originate in embryonic or germ cells may contain tissue of any or all of the possible cell types. *Anaplasia* is a change in the structure of cells characterized by a loss of differentiation (primitive form).

> **a.** *Benign* neoplasms (tumors) are characterized as being localized, single masses of cells, which remain at their site of origin. They usually are less aggressive, slower growing, and often surrounded by a capsule of dense tissue. Benign tumors may become life threatening if they disrupt the normal functioning of a vital organ. Benign tumors are removed by burning, freezing, chemical obliteration, or surgical procedures.

> **b.** *Malignant* neoplasms (tumors) are defined by their potential to include surrounding tissue or to escape to a new site in the body. Metastasis is the process of spreading to a secondary site and is believed to occur through lymphatic and circulatory channels. The term cancer is used to describe a malignant neoplasm. The term *tumor* is used as a synonym for neoplasm. Cancer is treated with chemotherapy, surgery, or radiation therapy. Chemotherapeutic medications for cancer are known as antineoplastics.

Both neoplasms and hyperplasias produce masses, which may be discovered by palpation, inspection, or diagnostic imaging (X-ray, CT scan, etc.). Most neoplasms are classified according to the cell or tissue type they resemble. The suffix "*oma*" is often added to indicate an abnormal growth (i.e. fibroma). If a malignant neoplasm arises from *epithelial* tissue, it is named a *carcinoma*. *Sarcoma* is used to name a malignant neoplasm arising from *other than* epithelial tissue. There are several exceptions to this naming system, such as "hematoma" which is not a neoplasm but a collection of blood within a tissue. Tumors may be further classified according to their location (epithelioma, adenoma, lymphoma).

C. The Integumentary System

Although most skin diseases are not life threatening, they may be very upsetting to the patient because of the unsightly appearance many can cause. A disorder of the skin is known as **dermatosis,** and may be as simple as sunburn or as deadly as cancer. Inflammation of the skin is known as **dermatitis**. Some of the most common dermatological problems, which are not life threatening are acne, cuts, moles (nevi), warts (verruca vulgaris), abscesses, eczema, seborrhea, psoriasis, and various types of rashes. Those that are life threatening would include severe burns, extreme sloughing of portions of the epidermis (due to a drug reaction), and malignant melanomas. Since the skin is essential to contain body fluids and regulate body temperature, loss or destruction to large areas can be fatal.

1. **Skin Lesions** - A lesion is any measurable alteration from the normal composition of a tissue. Lesions are not necessarily a sign of disease. For example, a flat lesion is a freckle. Lesions may be elevated, such as warts (papule), acne (pustule), insect bite (hive), burn or blister (vesicle), or psoriasis (plaque). Depressed lesions form a crack or break in the epidermis, such as a laceration, ulcer (bedsore), or Athlete's Foot (fissure). Skin lesions may also be an important indicator of a systemic disease; i.e., a red rash over both cheeks and the bridge of the nose is very common in patients with systemic lupus erythematosis and is often the first sign of the disease. Small, soft papules are common on the face and extremities of persons with elevated plasma lipid levels.

2. **Burns** - Burns are one of the most serious and frequent problems that affect the skin. Fire, contact with a hot surface, overexposure to sunlight, contact with an electrical current, or a harmful chemical can cause burns to the skin. The possibility for recovery depends on the total surface area involved. Burns are classified as:

   a. *First-degree* - Only some reddening of the skin will occur on the surface layers of the epidermis. Minimal pain is present.

   b. *Second-degree* - Causes damage to the deep epidermal layers and always to the upper layers of the dermis causing blistering, severe pain, swelling, fluid loss, and scarring.

   c. *Third-degree* - Complete destruction of the epidermis, dermis, and may involve underlying muscle and bone. Fluid loss is an extremely serious problem. Third degree burns may require reconstructive surgery.

3. **Skin Infections** - Skin infections occur when a virus, bacteria, fungus, or parasite invades this protective barrier. Examples of skin infections include:

a. Bacterial Skin Infections

1) Impetigo - A highly contagious condition most often occurring in young children. This can result from a staphylococcal or streptococcal infection. Beginning as a reddish discoloration (erythema), it soon develops vesicles and yellow crusts. If systemic, it may become life threatening. Impetigo is commonly treated with topical and/or oral antibiotics.

2) Furuncle *(Boil)* - Acute, tender, inflamed nodule around the hair shaft caused by the staphylococcal bacteria. Treated with hot compresses, possibly incision & drainage, and/or oral antibiotics.

3) Carbuncle - A cluster of furuncles that have spread deep beneath the epidermis. Treatment is the same as for furuncles.

4) Folliculitis - Infection of hair follicle, usually by the staph aureus bacteria. Treated with topical and/or oral antibiotics.

5) Cellulitis - Widespread infection caused by the streptococcus bacteria. Usually involves the skin and possibly deeper tissues, producing intense symptoms of inflammation without necrosis. *Erysipelas* - Superficial cellulitis with lymphatic involvement. Treatment is with IV and/or oral antibiotics.

6) Acne - Infection of the pilosebaceous glands by opportunistic skin bacteria causing inflammation and pus formation. Increased incidence during adolescence due to an increase in amount of sebum produced. Comedones (blackheads) are often present. Treatment is with antibacterial soaps, topical retinoic acid creams, oral antibiotics, oral retinoids, and dermabrasion for scarring.

7) Rosacea - Chronic inflammatory disorder, characterized by telangiectasia, erythema, papules, and pustules primarily on the central areas of the face. Cause is unknown, but it is more common in fair skinned people. Treatment is with metronidazole gel, oral antibiotics, or oral retinoids.

b. Viral Skin Infections

1) Fever Blisters *(Herpes Simplex 1 & 2)* - Contagious, painful, infection of herpes virus causing lesions around the mouth, on the lips, on the conjunctiva & cornea, and on the genitalia. Usually manifest in times of stress. Treatment is with systemic antiviral medications (Acyclovir, etc.).

2) *Shingles* *(Herpes Zoster)* - Contagious viral infection of dorsal nerve root ganglia, which causes inflammation in a dermatomal pattern. Treatment is with cool compresses, analgesics, and systemic antiviral medications (Acyclovir, etc.).

3) *Warts* *(verrucae)* - Contagious viral infection of epidermal cells causing mutation and hyperplasia. Different varieties may be found on all body surfaces. Treatment varies; most lesions disappear spontaneously within 2 years, but some may require topical ablation by the use of salicylic acid, lactic acid, retinoid cream, liquid nitrogen, laser therapy, electrodessication, or surgery.

4) *Pityriasis Rosea* - A mild inflammatory skin disorder characterized by scaly lesions and a self-limiting course. It is thought to be caused by a virus. Treatment if necessary, is with a topical (mild) corticosteroid cream.

c. *Fungal Skin Infections (Tinea)* - A broad term for many different types of opportunistic fungal (dermatophyte) infections of the skin. Tinea is characterized by erythema, scaling, and crusting. Sometimes fissures will develop in creases of the epidermis. Most are treated with topical antifungal creams, lotions, sprays or powders (miconazole, clotrimazole, ketoconazole, terbinafine, etc.). Some infections require a prolonged course of oral (systemic) antifungal medications (fluconazole, etc.).

1) *Tinea corporis* - Ringworm, *(Tinea capitus)* on the head
2) *Tinea pedis* - Athlete's Foot
3) *Tinea cruris* - Jock Itch
4) *Tinea versicolor* - Sun spots (loss of skin pigment)
5) *Tinea unguium* - Nail fungus
6) *Tinea barbae* - Barbers Itch (Ringworm of the beard)
7) *Candidiasis* (monoliasis) - Yeast infection that produces red patchy rash in skin folds and moist areas. Also produces white lesions on mucous membranes (mouth, vagina, etc.)

d. *Parasitic Skin Infections*

1) *Scabies* - Infection of the "itch mite" which burrows under the epidermis causing characteristic linear lesions and intense itching. It is transmitted by direct contact. Treatment is with a topical scabicide medication. Prednisone may be used for the itching.

2) *Pediculosis* *(lice)* - Infestation of small parasite causing inflammation and itching. Various forms prefer different areas of the body (head, body, groin). Treatment is with a topical pediculocide medication (permethrin cream or shampoo).

e. *Hypersensitivity Reactions*

1) *Contact dermatitis* - Histamine mediated allergic response to a substance, which has come in direct contact with the skin (poison ivy, jewelry, soap, cosmetics, etc.). Treatment includes avoidance of the offending substance and the use of either a topical or oral corticosteroid medication (prednisone).

2) *Atopic dermatitis* (eczema) - Chronic crusting, itching, and eruptions occurring primarily on flexor surfaces (knees, elbows, and other areas). Cause is often unclear, although allergic, hereditary, and psychogenic factors may be involved. Treatment includes avoidance of the offending substance and the use of either topical or oral corticosteroid medication (prednisone). Lubricating oils, antihistamines, and ultraviolet light therapy are also used.

3) *Seborrheic dermatitis* - Chronic inflammation characterized by redness, itching, dry/moist or greasy scaling, and yellow crusty patches on various areas, commonly including the face, ears, and scalp. It may be caused in part by the action of yeast on skin oils. Treatment includes the use of a topical antifungal creams or shampoos (zinc pyrithione, selenium sulfide, sulfur, coal tar), and a topical corticosteroid medication (prednisone).

4) *Hives* (wheals, urticaria) - Local histamine-mediated erythema, edema, and itching of the superficial dermis, due to drug allergy, insect bite/sting, or food allergy (eggs, shellfish, nuts, strawberries). Treatment is usually with oral antihistamines. *Angioedema* is characterized by deeper swelling and may involve the respiratory membranes. Treatment includes antihistamines and epinephrine.

f. *Neoplasms/Hyperplasias*

1) *Angioma* - A localized vascular lesion, resulting from hyperplasia of superficial blood vessels (port wine stain, vascular spider, strawberry birth mark). Treatment is with laser surgery.

2) *Lipoma* - Benign, soft movable, subcutaneous nodule composed of fat cells and enclosed in a fibrous capsule. Treatment if needed, is surgical excision or liposuction.

3) *Nevus* (mole) - A circumscribed malformation of the skin. May be pigmented and involve different types of cellular components (melanocytes, vascular elements, hair). Should be examined regularly for malignant changes. Treatment is surgical excision.

4) *Actinic Keratosis (liver spots, age spots)* - Circumscribed red or skin-colored lesion which may be pre-cancerous. Common on areas of skin that have received extensive exposure to U.V. light. Treatment if needed, is with topical retinoids, cryotherapy (liquid nitrogen), topical antineoplastics, or surgical excision.

5) *Seborrheic Keratosis* - Benign, usually pigmented, raised (wart-like) lesions, which often are soft, scaly, or waxy in nature. Treatment if needed, is with liquid nitrogen or surgical excision.

6) *Skin Tags* (Acrochordons) - Common, soft, pedunculated lesions, usually multiple, and occurring mainly on the neck, axilla, and groin. Treatment if needed, is freezing via liquid nitrogen, laser, or surgical excision.

7) *Sebaceous Cyst (keratin cyst or wen)* - Benign encapsulated tumor which contains keratin and sebum and forms a dense movable mass. Treatment is with surgical excision.

8) *Keloid Scar* - Smooth overgrowth of fibroblastic tissue arising at an area of injury. Keloids are more common in people of color. Treatment may include corticosteroid injections and surgery.

9) *Malignant skin tumors* - Occur in 50% of people age 65 or older. Most are on hands, head, and neck (areas of sun exposure). Major types include:

    a) Melanoma - 2% of skin cancer. 50% are lethal. Appear as raised or flat brown or black lesions with irregular borders and areas of different coloration (40-50% arise from a previously benign lesion such as a mole). Treatment is with aggressive surgical excision and chemotherapy.

    b) Basal Cell Carcinoma - Accounts for more than 50% of skin cancers. Slow growing, invasive lesions that may appear as firm raised nodules developing into ulcerated areas. Common in fair skinned people. Treatment (after biopsy) is with cryosurgery or surgical excision.

    c) Squamous Cell Carcinoma - Comprises 35% of skin cancers. Begins as a pigmented, scaly, plaque-like lesion that develops into an ulcerated crater. May be invasive. Common in fair skinned people. Treatment (after biopsy) is with cryosurgery or surgical excision.

g. *Miscellaneous Disorders of the Integumentary System*

1) *Comedone (blackhead)* - Dilated sebaceous gland, clogged w/ debris. Treatment is with antibacterial soaps, topical fruit acids, retinoic acids, and/or extraction.

2) *Eczema* - A general term like d*ermatitis*, and not a true diagnosis (see Contact Dermatitis). Characterized by chronic erythema, edema, vesicles, oozing, crusting, scaling, itching, and lichenification. Treatment is the same as for Contact Dermatitis.

3) *Lupus Erythematosis* - (SLE) Chronic, systemic, inflammatory disorder of connective tissue which often presents with a facial "butterfly" rash. Depending on the severity and manifestations, treatment may include the use of NSAIDs, antimalarial drugs, and/or immunosuppressive drugs (corticosteroids).

4) *Psoriasis* - Chronic, recurrent, inherited disorder characterized by the formation of silvery plaque-like scaly lesions occurring mainly on the extensor surfaces of elbows, knees, buttocks, and scalp. It may also be accompanied by a form of arthritis. Treatment may include the use of lubricating creams, topical corticosteroid medication (prednisone), anthralin /coal tar ointments, oral methotrexate, and/or psoralen-ultraviolet light (PUVA) therapy.

5) *Scleraderma* - Systemic, chronic, progressive disorder of the connective tissue, with an unknown etiology, characterized by thickening and hardening of the dermis (and internal organs). Treatment may include the use of oral immunosuppressive medications (prednisone, methotrexate), and vasodilators.

6) *Decubitus Ulcers* - (pressure sores, bed sores, trophic ulcers) Result from chronically decreased blood supply, usually from immobility, and often over a bony prominence. Treatment often involves topical wound care, topical antibiotics, hyperbaric oxygen therapy, PT, debridement, and plastic surgery.

D. The Skeletal System

Skeletal pathology is considered to include disorders of *Bone, Cartilage,* and *Ligamentous* structures. Fractures are by far the most common ailments of bone, yet if arthritis is considered a disease of the joints, then joint disease is much more common than bone disease. Sprains and strains are among the top causes for patients seeking health care for acute disease. Low back pain and degenerative arthritis rank high as causes for patients seeking treatment for chronic ailments. Metabolic disorders of skeletal system components also account for a large number of medical visits.

1. Structural Disorders

a. A *fracture* is a break or a rupture in a bone caused when the stress placed upon that bone exceeds its structural strength. Fractures may be the result of trauma alone or they may be *pathologic*, meaning that disease processes such as osteoporosis, cancer, or Paget's disease previously weakened the bone. The following terms are used to describe the characteristics of particular fractures:

1) An *incomplete* fracture produces cracks in a bone without entirely disrupting the continuity of the bone.

2) A *complete* fracture is one in which the bone is entirely separated into two or more pieces.

3) A *closed or simple* fracture does not produce an open wound in the skin.

4) An *open or compound* fracture is one in which the skin is broken.

5) A *comminuted* fracture is one in which the bone is splintered or crushed into more than two pieces.

6) A *compression* fracture is one in which the bone is pushed together by a compressive force rather than being broken apart.

7) The term *stress or fatigue* fracture refers to the accumulation of stress induced *micro fractures*, which may eventually result in a true fracture through the bone cortex.

8) A *greenstick* fracture is one in which one side of a bone is broken, the other side is bent.

9) A *fracture dislocation* is a fracture of a bone near a joint, also involving dislocation of that joint.

10) The term *nonunion* refers to the failure of a fracture to unite.

11) The term *malunion* refers to an unsatisfactory union of a fracture, with deformity in angulation, rotation, and length.

12) A *delayed union* fracture is one in which the union of bone takes a longer time than would be expected.

13) *Spiral, Oblique,* or *Transverse* describe the direction of break.

Location and *type* of fracture vary in frequency with sex and age, due to differences in activities leading to various types of injuries, and to the incidence of underlying disease. Traumatic fractures of the extremities are most common in 20 to 40 year old males, fractures of the clavicle and humerus are most common in children, and fractures of the hip and vertebrae are most common in elderly women as a result of increased osteoporosis.

Stress fractures are most common among athletes and frequently affect the long bones of the lower extremities, the calcaneus, and the second through fourth metatarsals. Fractures in general and Greenstick fractures in particular occur more frequently in children. Their bones are more flexible and less osteoporotic than adult bones. The humerus and clavicle are common fracture sites.

The most common *signs* and *symptoms* of a fracture include *pain* (often worse at night), *deformity, crepitus* (grating or crackling sound), *swelling*, and *muscle spasm* from adjacent muscular structures attempting to protect the damaged area. *Ecchymosis* or (bruising) discoloration of the surrounding tissue may also be present. Diagnosis is by X-ray.

Bones have a great capacity to heal. Continuity may be established in several weeks with a return to normal strength occurring in several months. The process of fracture healing involves the formation of a blood clot around the affected area, the formation of a callus or bony framework that stabilizes the bone fragments, and the process of remodeling, which is accomplished through the activity of osteoblasts and osteoclasts. Factors that affect bone healing include the proximity of the bone pieces, the presence of infection, the blood supply (and subsequent nutrition available), and the presence of an underlying disease. Fracture healing is much more rapid in the young than the elderly. Treatment usually involves casting (immobilization), buy may include surgical intervention, the use of pins, screws, plates, and bone grafts.

b. A *dislocation* or *luxation* is a displacement of a bone from its joint and usually involves damage to the joint capsule and surrounding ligaments. Occasionally the dislocation may include an injury to the articular surface and damage to the associated muscles and tendons. A *subluxation* is a partial or incomplete dislocation. The most common Signs and symptoms of a dislocation include deformity of the joint (may be fixed or locked in the deformed position), pain (worse by movement), and inability to use the joint (loss of function). Muscle spasm is common in surrounding tissues. Signs and symptoms of a subluxation might include joint deformity, pain, and joint dysfunction. Muscle spasm is also likely. Treatment usually involves manipulation and immobilization, but may require surgical intervention.

c. *Scoliosis* is a lateral curvature or deviation in the vertical line of the spine. *Congenital Scoliosis* is rare, but other vertebral anomalies are more common. *Idiopathic Scoliosis* is much more prevalent, occurring in about 4% of the population by 14 years of age. Sixty to 80% of cases occur in females. About one-half of those cases diagnosed require further treatment or follow-up. Signs and symptoms of scoliosis include postural abnormalities, fatigue in the lumbar area after prolonged standing or sitting, and pain or aching that becomes more persistent with continued irritation of the associated soft tissues. The prognosis is dependent on the severity and site of the curve. The greater the curve, the more likely there will be progression and complications. Prompt treatment is beneficial in limiting the progression of the condition and preventing further deformity. Treatment may involve exercise, yoga, electrical stimulation, osseous manipulation, corrective bracing, and/or surgery with (Harrington) rod insertion.

d. *Kyphosis* is the abnormally increased posterior convexity in the curvature of the thoracic spine as viewed from the side. Treatment may involve exercise/yoga, physical therapy, braces, and possibly surgery.

e. *Lordosis* is the abnormally increased anterior concavity of the lumbar spine. Both lordosis and kyphosis may be mild or severe, resulting from congenital abnormalities, spinal injury, or underlying disease. Complications of both may include loss of height and displacement of the internal organs. Deformations of other skeletal structures are a common occurrence as the body attempts to maintain its balance. Soft tissue structures such as muscle and ligament are often involved in these skeletal abnormalities. The prognosis for congenital abnormalities is poor, yet early treatment may limit the deformity. Conditions resulting from poor posture, weakened structural elements, and disease are more amenable to treatment. Treatment may involve exercise/yoga, physical therapy, and massage.

2. CONGENITAL, DEGENERATIVE, and DEFICIENCY DISORDERS

Diseases that directly affect bony structures include inherited disorders such as:

a. *Osteogenesis Imperfecta,* which reflects a defect in the development of all connective tissues, particularly of bone. This disorder is characterized by very thin, delicate, and abnormally curved bones, which lead to multiple fractures deformities. Fractures are often present at birth as are the characteristically blue sclera. Growth retardation, hearing loss, kyphoscoliosis, flat feet, and dental abnormalities are also common. Treatment usually includes physical and occupational theory. Drug therapy (biphosphates & calcitonin) for bone loss occasionally is used.

b. *Paget's Disease* or *osteitis deformans* is a condition caused by disordered bone remodeling, in which excessive bone resorption occurs and is followed by excessive and disorganized bone formation. This disease is relatively common, occurring in 3% to 4% of people over the age of 60 years. Northern Europeans have a high incidence of the disease, while in other groups the condition is almost nonexistent. The etiology of Paget's Disease is unknown, yet recent studies suggest that a virus may be involved. Signs and symptoms of this condition include *pain*, which may be related to micro-fractures, *thinning* and *thickening* of various portions of the skull, *deformities* of the facial bones, bone *tumors,* and circulatory changes leading to lightheadedness and possibly cardiac failure. Many patients with Paget's Disease are asymptomatic and require no treatment. Treatment for those with symptoms is palliative and includes NSAIDs, orthotics, and drug therapy (biphosphates & calcitonin).

c. *Osteoporosis* is characterized by loss of bone mass (including both collagen and minerals) due to a variety of conditions including decreased hormone production, reduced weight bearing activity, and insufficient levels of vitamin D or Calcium. Postural changes are common as well as fractures from bone weakening. Treatment includes hormone replacement therapy (HRT), calcitonin & biphosphates, exercise, and diet.

d. *Osteomalacia* or *Rickets* (in children) is characterized by softening of bone and loss of mass, due to a lack of vitamin D. It is common in developing nations but relatively rare in the U.S. Treatment (when adequate calcium is present) is with vitamin D.

e. *Ankylosing Spondylitis* is a chronic, systemic, inflammatory condition that leads to calcification and fusion of the spinal joints (often hip & low back). Other tissues including the eyes, lungs, kidneys, and heart may be effected. Treatment includes NSAIDs, oral corticosteroid drugs, physical therapy, exercise, and occasionally surgery.

f. *Spondylosis* is a term used to describe osteoarthritis of the spine. Treatment options include NSAIDs, oral corticosteroid drugs, physical therapy, exercise, and occasionally surgery.

g. *Spondylolisthesis* involves forward displacement of one vertebral body over another. The condition usually involves the lower lumbar region and often creates instability in that area. Treatment usually includes physical therapy, specific therapeutic exercise, and occasionally surgery.

h. *Chondromalacia Patella* involves deterioration of the articular cartilage on the posterior patella, causing pain and crepitus with forceful extension of the knee. Treatment includes non-weight bearing, repetitive exercise such as bicycling, avoiding weight bearing activity, and surgery.

3. INFLAMMATORY DISORDERS

a. *Osgood-Schlatter Disease* is characterized by ischemic necrosis of the tibial tuberosity leading to pain and swelling at the site of insertion of the patellar ligament. Common in children ages 10 to 15 years where calcification of the tibial tuberosity is incomplete. Treatment usually involves stretching and the avoidance of sport and excessive activities. Occasionally hydrocortisone injections and casting might be employed.

b. *Legg-Calve-Perthe Disease* involves aseptic, ischemic necrosis of the head of the femur. The disease is most common in children ages 5 to 10 years, the etiology is uncertain. Treatment may involve bed rest, traction, and immobilization via splints and/or casts.

c. *Osteomyelitis* is usually a bacterial (staph, strepp, tubercular) or fungal infection of the bone and marrow. Causes inflammation, necrosis, and destruction of bone. Treatment is with antibiotics, and may occasionally require surgical intervention.

d. *Bursitis* is inflammation of bursa from trauma, infection, or autoimmune disease. Treatment for uncomplicated cases may include NSAIDs, hydrotherapy, hydrocortisone injections, and surgery.

e. *Arthritis* - Joint inflammation
    1) *Osteoarthritis (DJD, osteoarthrosis)* - Most common of the arthritic diseases, resulting in degeneration of the articular cartilage & bony portions of a joint, and formation of bone spurs. It is usually a non-inflammatory condition thought to be caused by over-use. Treatment is with nonsteroidal anti-inflammatory drugs (NSAIDs), exercise, ROM activities, hyaluronic acid injections, corticosteroid injections, and occasionally surgery.

    2) *Rheumatoid Arthritis* - A chronic, systemic, inflammatory disease in which antibodies are produced in the synovial membrane of the joint capsule. Deformation of the joint is common. Treatment is with (NSAIDs), exercise & ROM activities, oral corticosteroids & methotrexate, and occasionally surgery.

    3) *Gout* - Chronic inflammatory condition caused by formation of uric acid crystals within the joint. Periods of remission and acute relapse are common. Treatment is with non-aspirin NSAIDs, steroidal anti-inflammatory drugs, increased fluid intake, weight loss & diet, and hypouricemic drugs (colchicine, allopurinol).

    4) *Lyme Disease* - A form of arthritis caused by bacterial infection brought about through a tick bite. Treatment is with antibiotics.

4. Miscellaneous Disorders

a. *Neoplasms* of the skeletal system are common and include such forms as the osteoma (benign), osteosarcoma (malignant), and the multiple myeloma (malignant). Treatment is as with other neoplastic disease.

b. *Sprains* are tearing injuries to the joint capsule or ligamentous structures. They can be painful and disabling. Sprains are graded as:
> *Grade One* - mild with 0-20% fiber tear, holds against resistance and perform normal motion, may be tender & swollen.
> *Grade Two* - moderate with 20-75% fiber tear, will show increased laxity with moderate resistance, presents with some edema, and muscle splinting. Function is altered.
> *Grade Three* - severe with 75-100% fiber tear, unstable, painful to touch, function is significantly altered. A "snap" is often noted.

c. *Herniated Disc* - Condition (with or without trauma) in which the nucleus pulposus protrudes or ruptures through the annulus fibrosis into the extradural space. The protruding disc may compress the spinal nerve root, cord, or cauda equina. The most common disc herniations occur at the L-5, S-1, C-6 and C-7 levels. Progressive severities of herniation are described by the terms bulge, protrusion, extrusion, and rupture. Disc related pain might be local or referred. Paresthesia and anesthesia may also result. Conservative treatment includes manipulation, traction, specific exercise, PT modalities, sedatives, muscle relaxing drugs, direct injections, and surgery.

d. *Bunions* - (hallux valgus) Condition involving lateral deviation of the large toe. There may be a genetic predisposition, but misalignment of the large toe is preceded by a weakening and loss of the transverse (metatarsal) arch of the foot. Bunions can be very painful and develop thick calluses. A Taylor's Bunion (bunionette) affects the smallest toe. Treatment includes prescription orthotics, specific exercise & stretching, corticosteroid injection and surgery.

e. *Pes Planus* - (flat feet) Condition involving loss of the medial (longitudinal) and transverse arches of the foot. The condition may be predisposed by a Morton's foot (shorter hallux than 2nd toe). Treatment includes prescription orthotics, specific exercise & stretching, and surgery.

f. *Plantar Fasciitis* - Inflammation of the plantar fascia. Conditions involving loss of the medial (longitudinal) arch of the foot leads to stress and inflammation of the plantar fascia. It may lead to the development of a heel spur (at the posterior attachment of the plantar fascia). Treatment involves the use of proper footwear, orthotics, exercise & stretching, nighttime splinting, NSAIDs, corticosteroid injection, and surgery.

g. *Dupuytren's Contracture* - (palmar fasciitis) is the idiopathic progressive shrinking and thickening of the palmar fascia. It may be related to a previous trauma. Treatment is with PT, stretching, cortisone injections, collagenase (enzyme) injections, and surgical release.

h. *Carpal Tunnel Syndrome* - Set of signs and symptoms arising from compression of the median nerve at the carpal ligament. Usually includes numbness, paresthesia, and weakness in the palmar aspect of the thumb, the 2nd, 3rd, and radial aspect of the 4th digits. Subluxation, inflammation, edema, fibrosis, and overuse (repetitive stress injuries) are thought to be causal. Systemic disorders may be implicated. Treatment includes night-splinting, Vitamin B-6, NSAIDs, acupuncture, ergonomic adjustments, corticosteroid injections, and surgery.

i. *Ganglion Cysts* - Cystic swellings of the tendon sheaths and joint capsules filled with a viscous fluid. The cause is unclear, although some appear following trauma. Treatment includes watchful waiting, aspiration, corticosteroid injection, and surgery.

j. *TMJ Syndrome* - A collection of symptoms including malocclusion, bruxism, and subluxation. Associated symptoms can include headache, face and neck pain, ear pain, and cervical subluxation. Treatment includes PT modalities, massage, NSAIDs, bite plates/splints, and surgery.

E. The Muscular System

Most muscular disorders *(myopathies)* involve either muscle wasting *(atrophy)* or muscle *hypertonicity* (abnormal increase in muscle tone). Except for the results of infection and trauma, most muscular problems are associated with nervous system dysfunction. Muscle pain is known as *myalgia,* while muscle inflammation is known as *myositis.*

1. A *cramp (spasm)* is a painful, spasmodic, involuntary, sustained muscular contraction, and may be a symptom of nerve irritation, ischemia, or an electrolyte (Na, K, Mg) and water imbalance. Treatment is fluid & electrolyte replacement.

2. *Tendinitis* is an inflammation of the tendon and/or tendon-muscle junction. *Tenosynovitis* includes inflammation of the tendon's synovial sheath. Both are commonly caused by repeated or extreme stress. Treatment includes R.I.C.E., PT modalities, local analgesic drugs, NSAIDs, hydrocortisone injections, surgery.

3. An *adhesion* is the abnormal joining together by collagen of two structures, commonly initiated by an inflammatory condition. Treatment is the prevention of inflammation, PT, massage, and ROM activity later in sub-acute stage.

4. A *contracture* is muscle tissue chronically shortened and resistant to passive stretching (as in Torticolis or "Wry Neck" w/ lateral flexion & rotation, which may involve SCM, Scalenes, or Upper Trapezius). May be due to scarring & fibrosis of muscle/supporting tissues, infections, tumors, or congenital deformities. Treatment includes PT modalities, massage, local analgesic drugs, NSAIDs, hydrocortisone injections.

5. *Strains* result from traumatic injuries to a muscle or tendon and are graded accordingly as:
   a. *First Degree* - mild with 0-10% fiber tear, usually has no palpable defects. Mild pain at time of injury, with increased tenderness and swelling later. Normal function is not compromised.
   b. *Second Degree* -moderate with 10-50% fiber tear, significant pain, some edema, and muscle splinting. Function is compromised.
   c. *Third Degree* - severe with 50-l00% fiber tear, unstable, edema, very painful, function significantly altered, the lesion or tear can be palpated, and a "snap" is often noted.

6. *Fibromyalgia* is a disorder characterized by symptoms of diffuse chronic (3 months minimum) pain and fatigue, sleep disturbances, coldness of the extremities, headaches, global anxiety, irritable bowel, and the presence of at least 11 "tender points." The cause is unknown. Treatment includes gentle massage, stress reduction, diaphragmatic breathing, and tricyclic antidepressant drugs.

7. *Chronic Fatigue Syndrome* is often associated with fibromyalgia and presents with generalized fatigue. May be linked to infection by the Epstein-Barr virus. Treatment involves healthful diet and lifestyle changes, massage, and a regimen of immune suppressant drugs and low-dose tricyclic antidepressants.

8. *Muscular Dystrophy* is a group of *genetic* diseases characterized by atrophy of skeletal muscle. The most common form is Dunchenne Muscular Dystrophy. Some forms of muscular dystrophy are fatal. Treatment involves genetic counseling, massage, PT, possibly surgery, and palliative care.

9. *Myasthenia Gravis* is a chronic disease characterized by muscle weakness that begins in the facial region and spreads to other skeletal muscle. It is an *autoimmune* disease and death results from respiratory failure. Treatment is similar to that for muscular dystrophy.

10. *Muscle infections* are caused by several microbes (bacteria, virus, or parasites) that produce muscle inflammation (*myositis*) or by underlying autoimmune disease. The muscular aching of influenza is a common example. Treatment is with rest, appropriate antimicrobial drugs (antibiotics, etc), or immunosuppressive drugs (if autoimmune).

11. *Chronic Myofascial Pain* - (MPS) is often associated with a cycle of ischemia-necrosis-pain, leading to continued contractions that produce further ischemia. Trigger points are common. Treatment involves trigger point therapy (spray & stretch, injections, or digital pressure), massage, and ergonomic changes.

12. *Whiplash* - Cervical Acceleration-Deceleration (CAD) is a broad term used to describe any number of soft tissue ailments usually associated with a rear impact auto accident. Treatment involves brief stabilization, (cervical collar), treatment for inflammation (RICE, anti-inflammatory drugs, PT modalities, etc.), ROM, therapeutic exercise, and massage.

13. *Thoracic Outlet Compression Syndromes* - Occurs when the neurovascular bundle (Brachial Plexus and/or Axillary Artery and/or Subclavian Vein) is compromised (entrapped) via Scalenus Anticus Syndrome, Cervical Rib Syndrome, and Shoulder Girdle Syndrome. Symptoms include pain and paresthesia in the hand, neck, shoulder or arms. Symptoms may be caused by a cervical rib, hypertonic scalenes, hypertonic pectoralis minor, or other dysfunction. Treatment depends upon cause, but may include massage, stretching and exercise, trigger point therapy, or surgery to remove the cervical rib.

14. *Hernia* - Refers to a "hole" through which constrained contents are escaping. They may be caused by congenital weakness, childbirth, or increased abdominal pressure. Hernias may be epigastric, paraumbilical, femoral, or inguinal. Treatment is with surgery to repair the tissue and inset mesh reinforcement.

F. The Nervous System

Diseases of the nervous system may affect any of the components including the brain, spinal cord, and the peripheral nerves. The major disease processes affecting the brain include *cerebrovascular accidents* (strokes), *traumatic injuries*, *infections*, and *neoplasms* (strokes being the third leading cause of death in the U.S). Headaches effect a large number of the population and degenerative diseases such as senile dementia, Alzheimer's, and Parkinson's are increasingly prevalent. Peripheral nerve disorders, such as herpes zoster and neuralgia, represent a significant number of medical complaints each year. Although not always associated with a disease of the nervous system, psychiatric (mental) disorders are also discussed in this section.

1. Central Nervous System

The most common symptoms of CNS disorders include headache, sensory loss, diminished motor functions, seizures, and changes in mental capabilities.

  a. *A.L.S.* (Amyotrophic Lateral Sclerosis, aka: Lou Gherig's Disease) A progressive, degenerative disease of motor neurons leading to muscle wasting and death. Cause is thought to be autoimmune. Treatment includes PT to maintain function, and palliative drug therapy.

b. *Alzheimer's Disease* - A specific type of senile dementia with characteristic lesions of the central cortex. The cause is unknown. Symptoms often include disorientation, irritability, and loss of memory for recent events. Treatment includes cholinesterase inhibiting drugs, NSAIDs, PT and OT to maintain function, and palliative drug therapy.

c. *Cerebral Palsy* - Permanent, non-progressive damage to motor areas of brain before or during birth from infection, trauma, hypoxia, or toxicity. Symptoms often include spastic paralysis. Treatment includes PT and OT to maintain function, and palliative drug therapy.

d. *Dementia* - Progressive degeneration of neurons in brain leading to personality changes, loss of memory, and diminished mental capabilities. Caused by trauma, infection (HIV, syphilis etc.), and unknown reasons. Care involves treating the underlying condition & palliative drug therapy.

e. *Encephalitis* - Inflammation of the brain. Viral infection is the most common cause (arbovirus via mosquitoes, poliovirus, coxsackievirus, HIV, herpes simplex, and others), but may follow acute lead poisoning or trauma. Treatment involves anti-viral drugs (Acyclovir), anti-inflammatory drugs (prednisone), and supportive therapy.

f. *Meningitis* - Infection/inflammation of the meninges with symptoms of fever, headache, stiff neck, malaise, and photophobia. Caused by bacterial, viral, fungal, and parasitic organisms. Treatment is with the appropriate anti microbial drug (antiviral, antibiotics, antifungal, etc), anti-inflammatory drugs (prednisone), and supportive care.

g. *Headaches* - Categorized as:
  1) *Vascular*
       a) **Migraine** (classic w/ aura or variant)
       Treatment includes avoidance of triggers (alcohol, cheeses), and vasoconstrictive drugs (cafergot, imitrex, Beta-blockers & Calcium channel blockers for prophylaxis)
       b) **Cluster** (similar to migraine, occur in clusters)
       Treatment is the same as for migraines
  2) *Tension* (decreased blood flow)
       Treatment include NSAIDs, tricyclic antidepressants, massage)
  3) *Cervicogenic* (trigger point referral)
       Treatment should address the underlying trigger points.
  4) *Chronic daily* (unknown or various etiologies)
       Treatment must be directed at suspected etiology.

h. *Huntington's Disease* -Inherited, progressive disorder causing uncontrolled muscular contractions (chorea). Onset is usually during the 30's and death occurs within 25 years. Treatment is the same as Dementia.

i. *Multiple Sclerosis* - Loss of myelin sheath covering neurons and plaque formation in CNS that decreases nerve conduction. Muscle wasting occurs. More common in women between ages of 20 and 40 years. Cause is unknown, but thought to be autoimmune. The disease has extended periods of remission followed by relapse. Treatment includes the use of corticosteroids, beta interferon, PT, and palliative therapy.

j. *Myelitis* - Infection/inflammation of a segment of the spinal cord. Treatment is non specific and symptomatic.

k. *Neoplasm* - Most CNS tumors are astrocytomas. Many other brain tumors are metastases from other areas of the body. Treatment involves chemotherapy, surgery and radiation.

l. *Neurofibromatosis* - Hereditary (genetic) disease characterized by multiple hyper-pigmented areas and numerous cutaneous & sub-cutaneous fibrous tumors, which arise from nervous tissue. Treatment involves genetic counseling, surgery, and radiation.

m. *Parkinson's Disease* - Chronic nervous disorder associated with degeneration of motor neurons of the mid-brain and decreases of a neurotransmitter. Symptoms include tremors at rest (pill- rolling), mask-like expression, and shuffling gait. Treatment involves Levo-dopa, antihistamines, antidepressants, MAO-B inhibitors, and PT.

n. *Seizure* - Abnormal neuron activity resulting in changes of consciousness, sensory perception, and motor control. May be mild or severe (convulsions). A condition of recurrent/chronic seizure episodes is known as Epilepsy. May be related to trauma, tumors, fever, or other causes. Treatment is anticonvulsive drugs, surgery, & ketogenic diet.

o. *Spina Bifida* - Failure of the dorsal structures to fuse during development including the vertebra. The spinal cord or meninges may be exposed. Treatment: adequate dietary Folate in pregnancy, or surgery.

p. *Stroke* - Cerebrovascular Accident (CVA) Death or dysfunction of neurons from ischemia. Brought about by a hemorrhage, thrombosis, or embolism. Symptoms often include paralysis, *paresis* (weakness), and *aphasia* (lack of ability to speak). Treatment: anticoagulant drugs.

q. *Transient Ischemic Attack* - (TIA) Vascular disturbance in brain tissue (with emboli), with stroke-like symptoms lasting less than 24 hours and followed by a complete recovery. Treatment may include anticoagulant drugs (heparin, warfarin, aspirin) and possibly bypass surgery.

2. Peripheral Nervous System

    a. *Bell's Palsy* - Inflammation of the *facial* (*7th cranial*) nerve. Symptoms include unilateral pain, numbness, and paralysis of face. Cause may be infection, immune dysfunction, or trauma. Treatment may include supportive care (natural/saline tears), electrostimualtion, and oral corticosteroid drugs early in the course of the disorder.

    b. *Carpal Tunnel Syndrome* - See condition under skeletal disorders.

    c. *Herpes Zoster/Shingles* - Infection of *spinal nerve* root and related *dermatome* by the latent (varicella) chicken pox virus. Usually occurs when the immune system is compromised. Symptoms include burning pain and a rash in a dermatomal pattern. Treatment is with cool-wet compresses, antiviral drugs (acyclovir, valacyclovir), oral corticosteroids, and topical capsaicin for pain of post herpetic neuralgia.

    d. *Neuralgia* - Nerve pain (see sciatica, etc.).

    e. *Neuritis* - *Inflammation* of the nerve (see herpes zoster, Bell's palsy).

    f. *Neuropathy* - Weakness, paresthesia, numbness, usually in distal area due to trauma or *degeneration* of peripheral nerve. Often a result of uncontrolled diabetes, heavy metal toxicity, vitamin B-6 toxicity, vitamin B-1 and B-12 deficiencies, and other chronic diseases. Treatment is directed to the underlying pathology.

    g. *Sciatica* - Pain, numbness, or tingling along the *sciatic nerve*. Cause may be trauma, infection, or compression (possibly by hypertonic *piriformis* or *bulging disc*). Treatment is directed to the underlying pathology.

    h. *Trigeminal Neuralgia* (Tic Douloureux) - Pain in the Trigeminal (*5th cranial*) nerve. Cause is unknown. Treatment includes the use of oral anti-seizure medications and possibly surgery for pain control.

    i. *Thoracic Outlet Syndrome* - see listing under muscular system.

3. Special Senses

    a. *The Eye:*

        1) *Astigmatism* - *Irregularity* in the shape of the lens or cornea. Treatment is with corrective lens.

2) *Cataract* - *Clouding* of the lens. Possibly from exposure to U.V. light. Treatment is corrective lens and ultimately surgery.

3) *Color Blindness* - *Genetic* defect in retina causing an inability to distinguish between one or more primary colors.

4) *Conjunctivitis (pink eye)* - *Inflammation* of the anterior conjunctiva. May be due to infection, allergy, or trauma. Treatment is generally topical and/or oral antibiotics, or antihistamines.

5) *Diabetic Retinopathy* - *Hemorrhage* in and *degeneration* of the retina. Major cause of blindness. Treatment is control of diabetes.

6) *Glaucoma* - Pressure of intraocular fluid is elevated. Second most common cause of blindness in US. Treatment is with topical or oral glaucoma drugs, laser, or surgery.

7) *Hyperopia* - Farsightedness is inability of the lens to focus on near objects. Treatment is with corrective lens or surgery.

8) *Myopia* - Nearsightedness is inability of the lens to focus on far objects. Treatment is with corrective lens or surgery.

9) *Nyctalopia* - Night blindness from *degeneration* of the retina or lack of vitamin A. Treatment is directed to pathology.

10) *Presbyopia* - Farsightedness of aging. Treatment is with corrective lenses.

11) *Strabismus & Amblyopia* (crossed-eyes) - Occurs when the positioning of the eyes is not coordinated. Treatment is with eye exercises, correctives lenses, and/or surgery.

12) *Hordeolum (stye)* - Acute localized infection of the gland(s) of the eyelash follicle. Reoccurrence is common. Treatment includes hot compresses, local and/or oral antibiotics.

b. *The Ear:*

1) *Meniere's Disease* - Chronic *inner ear* disorder of unknown origin. Symptoms include tinnitus, vertigo, and hearing loss. Treatment may include anticholenergic drugs (scopolamine), antihistamines, and surgery.

2) *Otitis Externa* - Inflammation of *external ear* often with symptoms of pain and redness. Treatment is with eardrops (vinegar and alcohol mixture), topical antibiotics, and dry heat.

3) *Otitis Media* - Inflammation of *middle ear,* often with symptoms of a deep ear ache pain. Treatment includes oral antibiotics, histamines, and avoidance of food allergens.

4) *Otitis Interna* - Inflammation of *inner ear,* often with symptoms of loss of balance and ringing in ear. Thought to be of viral origin. Treatment is the same as for Meniere's Disease.

5) *Tinnitus* - Ringing in the ear. Treatment is of the underlying cause, with a hearing aid, or with a sound-masking device.

6) *Vertigo* – Dizziness. A sense of spinning or moving around in space, associated with inner ear infection, toxemia, or tumor. Treatment may include manipulation, antihistamines, or otherwise be directed toward the underlying cause.

4. Mental Disorders: The major mental or psychiatric illness classifications include:

a. *Affective Disorders* - Characterized by alterations of mood; i.e. mania, depression and bipolar disorders. Treatment is with psychotherapy, behavior therapy, anti-depressant (heterocyclics, tricyclics, MAOIs, SSRIs, 5-HT agonists, etc), lithium carbonate, and anti-psychotic drugs

b. *Anxiety Disorders* - Characterized by neurotic symptoms such as panic attacks, phobias, and obsessive/compulsive behavior. Treatment is similar to that for affective disorders.

c. *Organic Disorders* - Dementia or illness due to diseases of the brain. See dementia for treatment information.

d. *Personality Disorders* - Life-long patterns of behavior that are unacceptable with regard to accepted social norms (borderline, antisocial, narcissistic, dependent, passive-aggressive, etc.). Treatment usually involves prolonged psychotherapy. Drug therapy has limited effects.

e. *Schizophrenia* - A thought disorder leading to misinterpretation of reality. Often includes delusions and hallucinations. Treatment includes the long-term use of anti-psychotic drugs (Fluphenazine, Haloperidol).

G. The Endocrine System

The endocrine system is responsible for the regulation of ongoing physiological functions (homeostasis). A dysfunction in this system usually causes a chronic disorder affecting many body parts. There are many types of endocrine system diseases and most result from either a hyposecretion or a hypersecretion of hormones. The faulty production of hormone may be triggered by infection, autoimmune disease, or trauma. There may also be problems raised by an insensitivity of the target organ to its controlling hormone. Only the most common of endocrine system disorders are discussed here. *Treatment might include the replacement of the deficient hormone, supplementing vital nutrients, (Iodine, Vit. K, etc), or ablation of the overactive gland (via surgery or radiation).*

1. Pituitary - *Hyposecretion* influences many other endocrine gland functions in that the pituitary functions as the "Master Gland." Too little pituitary hormone may cause diabetes, hypothyroidism, dwarfism or lack of sexual development. *Hypersecretion* could conversely be responsible for giantism or acromegaly, hyperthyroidism, and abnormal water retention.

2. Thyroid - *Hypothyroidism* (from multiple causes) symptoms: weight gain, lethargy, coldness, dry skin / hair, constipation, and depression. *Hyperthyroidism*, (from multiple causes) symptoms: tachycardia, weight loss, anxiety, restlessness, insomnia, increased temperature, increased perspiration, and exophthalmia.

3. Parathyroid - *Hyposecretion* results in low blood levels of calcium and possibly muscle contraction problems. *Hypersecretion* may cause a high level of blood calcium and thus calcification of muscle and other inappropriate tissues.

4. Adrenal - *Hyposecretion* may cause Addison's Disease and dehydration. *Hypersecretion* may result in Cushing's Syndrome and increased water retention.

5. Pancreas - There are two or more types of diabetes mellitus (meaning sweet urine) characterized by hyperglycemia (fasting blood sugar ≥ 140). Type 1 DM is also known as "insulin dependent" or juvenile onset. The cause is autoimmune with resulting destruction (90% or more) of the Beta cells of the pancreas and an inability to produce insulin. Type 2 DM usually occurs after the age of 30, and may involve decreased insulin secretion or insulin resistance. Common symptoms are polyuria, polydipsia, and polyphagia. Complications are cardiovascular disease, peripheral vascular disease w/ peripheral neuropathy, kidney disease, blindness and increased infections. Type 1 DM requires insulin therapy. Type 2 DM may be treated with diet, exercise and oral hyperglycemic medications. Gestational DM is diabetes of pregnancy. *Hypersecretion* of insulin causes decreased blood sugar levels (hypoglycemia) and may be fatal (insulin shock).

6. Ovary/Teste - Abnormal production of sex hormones causes either premature or lack of development of secondary sexual characteristics.

7. Thymus -*Hyposecretion* produces a depression of the immune system.

8. Pineal - H*ypersecretion* of hormone produces "seasonal affective disorder" (winter depression). May be involved in sleep disorders.

H. The Circulatory System - Blood & Lymph

Various disorders beset the heart and vessels, ultimately interrupting the flow of blood to cells, resulting in *hypoxia* (oxygen deficiency) or *anoxia* (no oxygen). Cell death *(necrosis)* occurs and tissue is damaged. As all cells in the human body are dependent upon the circulatory system for transportation, every system suffers when cardiovascular disease is present. Cardiovascular disease accounts for nearly 40% of all deaths in the U.S. The most common disorders are discussed:

1. *Myocardial Infarction (Heart Attack)* - Death of cardiac muscle cells from ischemia. Often caused by coronary thrombosis or arteriosclerosis. Treatment includes critical care (thrombolytic drugs - streptokinase, etc.), aspirin heparin, vasodilators, ACE inhibitors, B-Blockers, angioplasty, bypass surgery, followed by lifestyle modification, aspirin therapy, propranolol, and rehabilitation.

2. *Angina Pectoris* - Transient pain during exertion caused by ischemic cardiac muscle. Treatment includes lifestyle modification, hypertension medications, nitroglycerine, antiplatelet drugs (aspirin), angioplasty, and bypass surgery.

3. *Congestive Heart Failure* - Failure of the left side of the heart to pump effectively, resulting in congestion in the systemic and pulmonary circulatory systems. Treatment includes diuretics, Ace inhibitors, B-Blockers, Digitalis.

4. *Hypertension* - Elevation of systolic (>140) and diastolic (>90) blood pressure is of unknown etiology. Dietary Na, obesity and stress may contribute only in predisposed persons. Hypertension is asymptomatic until complications develop. These include heart failure, atherosclerosis, stroke, and retinal & kidney disease. Treatment includes diet (high in Ca, K, Mg and fiber) & exercise, diuretics, B-blockers, Ca blockers, ACE inhibitors, and Angiotensin inhibitors.

5. *Arrhythmia* - Abnormal heart rate. Treatment is anti-arrhythmia drugs.

6. *Rheumatic Fever* - Cardiac damage from inflammatory response to a bacterial infection. Treatment is aspirin and antibiotics.

7. *Heart Murmurs* - Abnormal heart sounds caused by disorders of the valves.

8. *Aneurysm* - Weakening and widening of an artery wall. Tendency to rupture and form clots. Treatment is hypertension medication and surgical resection.

9. *Varicosity* - Weakening and widening of vein wall, with a tendency to form clots. Treatment is with exercise, compression clothing, injection therapy, and surgery.

10. *Thrombophlebitis* - A clot in a vein with inflammation. Treatment is with NSAIDs, hot compresses, heparin, urokinase, and support hose (with edema).

11. *Anemia* - Inability of red blood cells to deliver enough oxygen to tissues producing symptoms of fatigue. Treatment involves supplementing the deficient red blood cell component (Iron, B-12, Folate, Copper, Vit C, protein), treating the underlying pathology (blood loss, bone marrow disorder, chronic disease, autoimmune disease), or congenital RBC defects (Sickle cell, Thalassemias).

12. *Hemophilia* - Genetic inability to form blood clots and, therefore, to control bleeding. Treatment is transfusion of plasma or clotting factors (VIII or IX).

13 *Edema* - Presence of abnormally large amounts of fluid in the interstitial tissue spaces. May be caused by increased capillary pressure, reduced plasma protein, or increased intracellular sodium. (*Pitting edema* is characterized by indentations that remain for a time after pressure is released; may result from prolonged sitting or standing, or venous dysfunction.) Treatment is directed toward underlying pathology (hypertension, CHF), support hose, and diuretics.

14. *Allergy* - Hypersensitivity to normally harmless environmental substances with formation of an antigen that can lead to an inflammatory response (types I thru IV). Treatment involves identifying and avoiding the offending agents, desensitization therapy, oral & topical antihistamines, and immediate injection of epinephrine in anaphylaxis.

15. *Hepatitis* - A general description for inflammation of the liver. May be caused by excessive alcohol consumption (leading to fibrosis or cirrhosis), viral infection (hepatitis A, B, C, D, E, and G), and drug toxicity (acetaminophen, MAOIs, isoniazid, and halothane). Treatment may involve avoidance of the toxic material, supportive care, and the drugs interferon & ribavirin (for B & C).

16. *HIV/AIDS* - HIV is a viral infection with the human T-cell HIV-1 or HIV-2 viruses. HIV is both oncogenic and lymphotrophic. HIV may be transmitted via any body fluid that contains plasma or lymphocytes, specifically blood, semen, vaginal secretions, breast milk, saliva, and wound exudates. HIV is not transmitted by "casual" contact. The presence of other sexually transmitted diseases increases the rate of HIV transmission. AIDS is a disorder of cell-mediated immunity characterized by opportunistic infections, malignancies, neurologic dysfunction, and a variety of other syndromes. The progress of AIDS presents with a predictable pattern. *Phase 1* (averages 3 weeks to 6 months) is asymptomatic, with an increasing viral load and high potential for transmission. In *Phase 2*, HIV antibodies become detectable, and for a short (2 week) duration, fatigue, lymphadenopathy, fever, headache, weight loss, drowsiness and other flu-like symptoms are noted. *Phase 3* involves the asymptomatic (controlled) replication of the virus. This phase may last from 1 to 15 years (10 years is average), depending on the victim's general health. Symptoms of AIDS appear in *phases 4 and 5*. Symptoms commonly include Pneumocystis carnii, Karposi's sarcoma (skin cancer), Cytomegalovirus infection (retinitis, colitis, etc), Non-Hodgkin's lymphoma, toxoplasmosis, herpes (simplex & zoster), candidiasis, and tuberculosis. Treatment includes antiviral drugs (HAART), and supportive therapy.

I. The Respiratory System

The respiratory system is quite susceptible to trauma from environmental pollutants (car exhaust, cigarette smoke, chemicals) as well as being exposed to a variety of infectious agents (bacteria, virus, and fungus). Acute respiratory disease is the leading cause of people seeking medical care. Lung cancer is responsible for over one-third of all cancer deaths. The respiratory system is divided into two major components—upper (above the larynx) and lower (below the larynx) with many conditions being described accordingly:

1. Upper Respiratory Tract Infections: May be of bacterial, viral, or fungal origin. The common cold is an example of a viral disorder, resulting in copious mucous discharge from mucous membranes. Diseases are described according to the area of infection. The following are common upper respiratory tract disorders:

> **a.** *Rhinitis* - Inflammation of the nasal mucosa, common cold (allergic, bacterial, viral). Treatment is primarily palliative (antihistamines, decongestants, vasoconstrictors, and antibiotics when appropriate).

> **b.** *Pharyngitis* - Common "sore throat" is usually viral, but could be bacterial or fungal. Treatment is acetaminophen, and antimicrobial drug.

> **c.** *Sinusitis* - Inflammation of the mucosa lining the sinus cavities. May be viral, bacterial, fungal or allergic. Treatment is saline irrigation, anti-histamines, vasoconstrictors, and antibiotics when appropriate.

2. Lower Respiratory Tract Infections:

> **a.** *Pleurisy* - Pleuritis, inflammation of the pleural membrane. May be a symptom of underlying disease or direct infection. Pain made worse by respiration/cough is key symptom. Treatment is for the underlying cause.

> **b.** *Bronchitis* - Inflammation of the bronchial tubes (may be acute or chronic in nature). Usually viral in nature. Treatment is rest, fluids, symptomatic care, and antibiotics when appropriate.

c. *Pneumonia* - Inflammatory condition of the lungs in which the airways become filled with thick fluid (*exudate*). Fever and productive cough are symptoms. Bacterial infection is the most common cause, although viral and fungal organisms are implicated. Treatment is antimicrobial drugs.

d. *Tuberculosis* - Chronic, contagious, mycobacterial infection causing fatigue, weight loss, chest pain, and fever. The infective agent may spread from the lungs to other tissues. Number of cases has greatly increased in recent years. Treatment is with long-term antibiotic therapy.

e. *Asthma* - An obstructive disorder characterized by recurring spasms of the smooth muscle in the bronchi, obstruction, inflammation, and increased mucous secretion. Asthma is characterized by expiratory wheezing. The cause is not well understood but the disease may be triggered by stress, exercise, or allergies. Treatment involves avoidance of known allergens, anti-inflammatory (corticosteroid) drugs, and both short & long term bronchiodilating drugs (B-adrenergics and theophylline).

f. *Emphysema* - COPD, The result of chronic trauma to lung tissue from smoking or exposure to other pollutants. The alveoli rupture and form large non-functioning spaces within the lungs. Hypoxia results from the reduced respiratory capacity. Treatment includes the cessation of smoking, bronchiodilator drugs (albuterol, etc), theophylline, corticosteroids, antibiotics, increased hydration (to thin sputum), and oxygen therapy.

J. The Digestive System

The digestive system combines many types of tissue and is susceptible to various disorders. Only the most common diseases will be discussed.

1. *Oral Cancer* - More common in those who smoke or chew tobacco and in regular alcohol users. These constitute 5% of all cancers in the U.S. The lesions often appear as a chronically inflamed area. Treatment is surgery or radiation.

2. *Apthos Ulcers (canker sores)* - Painful ulcers affecting the oral mucous membrane. They may last from days to weeks. The cause is unknown, but they are suspected of being an autoimmune disorder. Stress and trauma appear to be related factors. Treatment involves local anesthetics and corticosteroids.

3. *Glossitis* - Inflammation of the tongue usually associated with chronic disease (Vit B-12, Iron deficiency). Treatment is directed at the underlying pathology.

4. *Hiatal Hernia* - Condition in which the superior portion of the stomach ascends through the cardiac sphincter of the diaphragm. Symptoms of heartburn are common (which are made worse by lying down). Treatment is generally symptomatic (antacids and H_2 Blockers), but may include surgery.

5. *Esophagitis* - Inflammation of the esophagus caused by gastric reflux (GERD), bulimia, alcoholism, or other factors. Esophagitis may also produce heartburn. Treatment is directed at the underlying pathology, and may include raising the head of the bed, avoidance of certain foods (coffee, alcohol, fats, chocolate), avoiding smoking, use of antacids, and H_2 Blockers.

6. *Peptic Ulcers* - Recurring ulceration of either the stomach (gastric) or the small intestine (duodenal). Risk factors include stress, cigarette smoking, alcohol consumption, and overuse of aspirin. Associated with bacterial (H. pylori) infection. Treatment includes antibiotics to eradicate H. pylori, H_2 Blockers, antacids, Proton Pump Inhibitors, dietary changes, and surgery.

7. *Crohn's Disease* (*regional enteritis*) - Characterized by inflammation of segments of the small or large intestine. Inflammation brings fibrous scar tissue formation that in turn makes the affected region of the bowel dysfunctional. Crohn's is progressive and often deadly. The etiology of Crohn's Disease is thought to be of a genetic and autoimmune nature. Treatment involves the use of muciloids (psyllium), corticosteroids, immunomodulating drugs, and surgery.

8. *Lactose Intolerance* - A genetically predisposed condition in which an insufficient amount of the carbohydrate-digesting enzyme (lactose) is made. The disease causes gas, bloating, pain, and diarrhea and affects specific ethnic populations (African, Asian, and Mediterranean). Treatment involves avoidance of lactose containing foods and/or supplementing the enzyme lactase.

9. *Cholecystitis* (acute gall bladder inflammation) - Chronic condition causing abdominal pain that is aggravated by fatty foods. More common in fair skinned, obese, women over the age of 40, with an American diet. *Cholelithiasis* is the formation of gallstones. Treatment is surgical removal of the gall bladder.

10. *Diverticulosis* - Presence of sac-like dilatations in the intestinal wall. Most are found in the distal large intestine. When the sacs become inflamed, the condition is known as *diverticulitis*. It is estimated that 50% of the U.S. population have diverticula. May be due to the low fiber, highly refined American diet. Treatment includes a high fiber (psyllium) diet, and surgery for cases that do not respond to conservative care.

11. *Irritable Bowel Syndrome* - (IBS) A condition of unknown cause, with pain, diarrhea, constipation, and bloating. Emotional stress, diet and hormones are thought to be associated factors. Treatment is supportive & palliative, and involves increased muciloids (psyllium), and avoidance of diary products, artificial sweeteners, high fructose foods and other food allergens.

12. *Polyps* - Outgrowths of tissue into the intestine. May be benign or malignant and should be biopsied. Treatment includes a high fiber (psyllium) diet, and surgery for cases that do not respond to conservative care.

13. *Stomach* **and** *Colon Cancer* - Are common diseases in developed countries where low-fiber diets are common. The first symptoms often include dysphasia, a sense of fullness, bleeding and changes in bowel habits. Treatment includes chemotherapy and surgery.

K. The Urogenital System

For convenience, disorders of the urinary and genital systems are discussed together. Bacterial infections are the most common ailment of the urogenital systems. Yet a wide variety of neoplasms are found in both males and females. Compared to other organ systems, congenital anomalies of the urogenital organs are relatively uncommon.

1. *Cystitis* (bladder infection) - More common in females due to easier access to the bladder by bacteria from the perineum. Pathogens (especially chlamydia) may also be sexually transmitted. The most common symptoms of cystitis include frequent urination, pain, and possibly low back pain. Where the urethra is inflamed (urethritis), burning with urination is present. Treatment involves forcing fluids and the use of antibiotics.

2. *Nephritis* (inflammation of the kidney) - Whether acute or chronic it is commonly bacterial in nature (usually E-coli) and results from movement of pathogens *up the urinary tract from the bladder and ureters*. Symptoms of nephritis include low back pain and significant numbers of protein, bacteria, and white and red blood cells in the urine. When a urinary obstruction exists, conditions persist as low-grade chronic infections despite treatment. Treatment is similar to that for cystitis.

3. *Prostatitis* - Acute or chronic inflammation of the prostate gland. Often bacterial in nature and may be a sexually transmitted disease. Symptoms often include pain and difficulty with urination. Treatment is the same as for cystitis.

4. *Prostatic Hypertrophy* (hyperplasia,) - May be either benign (BPH) or malignant and both are common and significant diseases of the elderly. Both diseases produce urinary problems and increased infections are common. Drugs to increase urine flow, radiation, and surgery are both used therapeutically, with impotence and/or incontinence often being side effects of radiation and surgery.

5. *Kidney Stones* (urolithiasis) - Most commonly formed of calcium and produce no symptoms until they attempt to pass down through the ureters. Symptoms include flank pain that radiates toward the groin and often hematuria (blood in the urine). Treatment involves narcotics, forcing fluid, lithortripsy (ultrasound), surgery, and identification of the offending stones to prevent recurrences.

6. *Vaginitis* (inflammation of the vaginal tissue) - Results from infection by bacteria (chlamydia, gonorrhea, syphilis), fungus (candida), virus (herpes), or parasite (trichamonas). Symptoms often include a vaginal discharge, pain or itching, and inflammation. If left untreated, it can spread to the fallopian tubes and ovaries. When the organism escapes the above organs, it is known as *Pelvic Inflammatory Disease (PID)*. Treatment is with the antimicrobial drugs.

7. *Ovarian Tumors* - Quite common and represent several different types of abnormal growths. Carcinoma of the endometrium is the most common. The primary symptom is bleeding, and therapy gives about an 80% survival rate. Fibroid tumors (Leiomyomas) are benign "space occupying" lesions that develop during the childbearing years. They are usually asymptomatic but may present with pelvic pressure, bleeding, or infertility. Diagnosed by exam and x-ray. (Carcinoma of the cervix is commonly diagnosed by the PAP test). Treatment involves hormone therapy, chemotherapy, and/or surgery.

8. *Endometriosis* - The presence of endometrial tissue outside the uterus. Symptoms include pain, excessive bleeding, and infertility. Treatment involves hormone therapy (OBC), pregnancy and/or surgery.

9. *Carcinoma of the Breast* - By far the most important breast disease. One out of every eight women develops breast cancer, and it is a significant cause of death. Other breast tumors need to be noted and differentiated from carcinoma. Fibrocystic disease accounts for most breast disease, and although benign, it may predict more serious tumor development. The most significant sign of a breast tumor is the detection of a lump. Treatment involves hormone therapy, chemotherapy, and/or surgery (lumpectomy thru radical mastectomy).

Review Question - Clinical Pathology

1. Which hypertonic muscle might result in rotation of the Ilium causing a functional short leg?
    a) Biceps femoris
    b) Iliopsoas
    c) Rectus abdominis
    d) Gluteus medius

2. Chronic inflammation and fibrosis of the rotator cuff musculature could result in:
    a) Hyper-mobility of the shoulder
    b) Antalgic gait
    c) Frozen shoulder
    d) Winged scapula

3. Because of their lack of vascularity, the following tissue is known to heal quite slowly:
    a) Epithelial
    b) Fibrous connective
    c) Muscle
    d) Bone

4. Inflammation of the bladder, most commonly caused by the presence of a pathogenic bacteria and leading to frequent urination is called:
    a) Nephritis
    b) Hepatitis
    c) Diverticulitis
    d) Cystitis

5. Warts are benign neoplasms that are due to infection by this contagious organism:
    a) Bacteria
    b) Fungus
    c) Parasites
    d) Virus

6. Inflammation of the appendix might present with pain in the:
    a) Upper right quadrant
    b) Lower left quadrant
    c) Lower right quadrant
    d) Upper left quadrant

7. Wasting of an organ or tissue from non use is known as:
    a) Hypertrophy
    b) Hematoma
    c) Crepitus
    d) Atrophy

8.   The state or condition in which the body or part of it are invaded by a pathogenic agent the multiplies and causes cellular injury is know as:
       a) Inflammation
       b) Induration
       c) Infection
       d) Infarction

9.   Inflammation is characterized by:
       a) Pain, tenderness, heat, and swelling
       b) Pain heat tenderness to touch, and swelling
       c) Heat, redness, swelling, and dryness
       d) Pain, heat, redness, and swelling

10.   A joint injury in which some of the fibers of the supporting ligament or joint capsule are damaged is known as:
       a) Subluxation
       b) Strain
       c) Sprain
       d) Dislocation

11.   The abnormal joining together of tissues after inflammation is known as:
       a) Adenoma
       b) Adhesion
       c) Inflammation
       d) Infection

12.   Abnormal extreme posterior curvature of the Thoracic Spine is commonly known as:
       a) Kyphosis
       b) Scoliosis
       c) Lordosis
       d) None of the above

13.   Soreness, numbness, and weakness of the hand due to compression of the Median nerve at the Flexor Retinaculum and Transverse Carpal Ligament is referred to as:
       a) Thoracic outlet syndrome
       b) Scalene syndrome
       c) Carpal tunnel syndrome
       d) Brachial plexus syndrome

14.   The chronic disease of the Liver, characterized by formation of dense connective tissue, resulting in loss of function and increased resistance to blood flow is:
       a) Hepatitis
       b) Cystitis
       c) Cholecystitis
       d) Cirrhosis

15. A condition caused by a break or leak in a blood vessel, resulting in a swelling and accumulation of blood within an organ, tissue, or space is known as a:
a) Hypertrophy
b) Abrasion
c) Hematoma
d) Adhesion

16. A partial or incomplete dislocation of a bone at an articulation is a:
a) Subluxation
b) Involution
c) Amphiarthrosis
d) Subinvolution

17. A decrease in blood flow to a tissue or organ, resulting in impairment of cell function or in cell death is known as:
a) Anemia
b) Aneurysm
c) Ischemia
d) Necrosis

18. An inflammatory disease of the skin involving sebaceous glands and hair follicles, and characterized by comedones, papules, and pustules is known as:
a) Psoriasis
b) Acne
c) Scabies
d) Decubitus ulcers

19. Protrusion of the stomach into the mediastinal cavity above the diaphragm is:
a) Hiatal hernia
b) Osgood-schlatter disease
c) Diverticulosis
d) Marfan's sydrome

20. A chronic degenerative joint disease characterized by deterioration of articular cartilage, overgrowth of bone, and impaired function is known as:
a) Gout
b) Rheumatoid arthritis
c) Osteoarthritis
d) Osteoporosis

21. This disease which is common among the elderly and is marked by a loss of bone mass and subsequent loss of bone strength is:
a) Chondromalacia patellae
b) Osteoporosis
c) Osteoarthritits
d) Lyme disease

22. The fungal infection of the skin which is characterized by whitish or fawn-colored irregular shaped patches is known as:
   a) Tinea pedis
   b) Tinea versicolor
   c) Tinea cruris
   d) Leprosy

23. Peripheral neuropathy and decreased arterial circulation in the extremities is associated with this degenerative disease:
   a) Sciatica
   b) Diabetes
   c) Rheumatoid arthritis
   d) Gout

24. A blood clot, which has recently formed in a varicose vein and is still stationary is known as:
   a) Embolus
   b) Thrombus
   c) Embolism
   d) Infarction

25. The weakening of the muscular portion of an artery that causes the vessel to dilate abnormally and potentially to rupture is:
   a) Aneurysm
   b) Varicosity
   c) Bypass
   d) Claudication

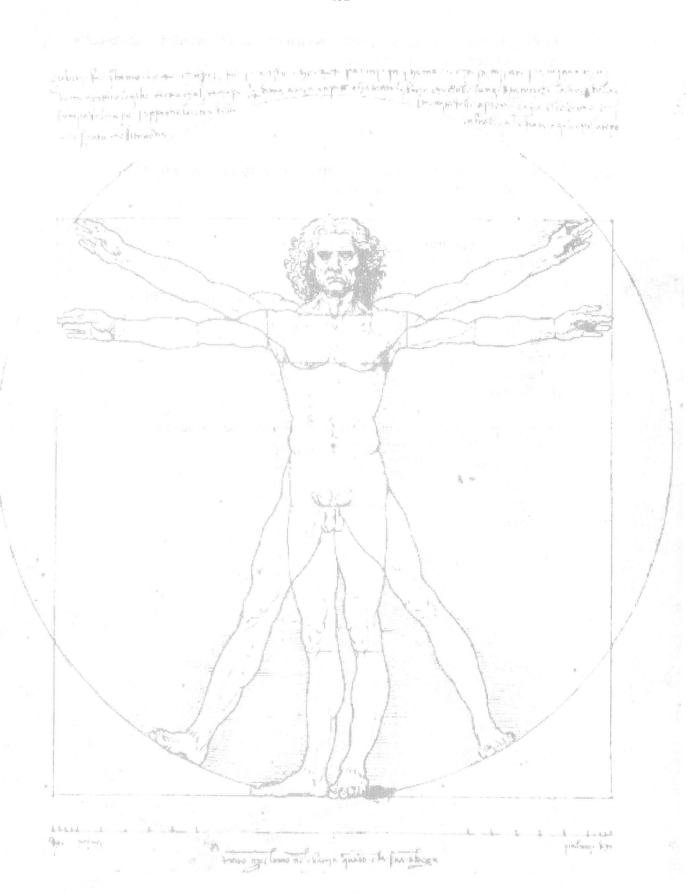

III-A. MASSAGE/BODYWORK THEORY, ASSESSMENT, AND PRACTICE

A. Definition

Massage is the intentional and systematic therapeutic manipulation of the human body's soft tissues. Massage Therapists manipulate the soft tissue using their hand, foot, arm, or elbow. Joint movements and stretching are often integrated into the practice of massage therapy. State laws may vary in their legal definitions of massage therapy.

B. History

Massage is an ancient remedy. The *History of Chinese Medicine* refers to acupuncture, moxa, and massage. As early as 3000 B.C., Chinese books described a massage technique called *Anma.* The early Indian medical writings, *Ayur-Veda*, mention massage. Greek and Roman gladiators used massage to relieve pains and bruises, and to invigorate the body. **Hippocrates** (400 B.C.) was one of the first to discuss the qualities and contraindications of massage. **Per Henrik Ling** of Sweden (1776-1839), a fencing master and instructor of gymnastics, is the father of Swedish Massage. Prominent contributors to the field include:

1. James Cyriax's, *Textbook of Orthopaedic Medicine, Vol. II* in 1977 describes a deep transverse friction technique that restores mobility to muscle. He emphasized slow and unidirectional stroking, even rhythm and light pressure, massaging the proximal limb before the distal. Deep transverse friction *broadens* the fibrous tissues of muscles, tendons, or ligaments, breaking down fibrous *adhesions* and restoring mobility.

2. Elizabeth Dicke in 1929 developed a system known as *Bindegewebsmassage,* a connective tissue massage technique. She discovered certain areas on the body relate to certain viscera, and that imbalance especially affects the autonomic and central nervous system.

3. Douglas Graham's, *Treatise on Massage, Its History, Mode of Application and Effects,* aroused the American medical profession's interest.

4. Albert J. Hoffa, German physician and author of the basic massage text, *Technik der Massage.* He used an anatomical method for dividing the body parts to be massaged. He did not advocate massage for any longer than 15 minutes.

5. Dr. John Harvey Kellogg, in 1895 wrote the first edition of *The Art of Massage* describing the scientific practice of massage at his Battle Creek Sanitarium. Considered by some to be the "consummate" book on massage.

6. Mary McMillan, Chief Aide at Walter Reed Army Hospital in 1918 and later Director of Physiotherapy at Harvard Medical School, had a background in massage and therapeutic exercise and wrote a basic text for physiotherapy. She divided massage into five basic strokes and defined the specific area to be massaged. In each area involved, the stroke is carried from just below the distal joint to just beyond the proximal joint, the object being to assist lymph flow back to the heart.

7. Johann Geog Mezger (1838-1909), a Dutch physician, classified soft tissue manipulations into four categories using the French terms *effleurage, petrissage, friction*, and *tapotement*.

8. Dr. M. Roth, a British physician published the first English language translation of Ling's system in 1851.

9. Harold D. Storms in 1944 published an article describing a diagnostic as well as therapeutic massage friction stroke (parallel to the muscle fibers).

10. Dr. George Taylor brought the "Swedish Movement Cure" to the United States in 1854.

Since the early 1980s, massage therapy has grown into a profession with national and state associations involved in legislation to enhance the image of the profession, as well as integrate this profession into the health care field.

C. Purpose

Massage physically increases cell metabolism, hastens healing, increases range of motion, and relieves pain. Psychologically massage may relieve fatigue, reduce anxiety and tension, and promote relaxation.

D. Effects on the Body

Mechanical effects result from the direct pressure of the massage techniques on the body. Compression of the tissue assists venous and lymphatic flow. Petrissage and friction disrupt adhesions. Assisted stretching techniques lengthen shortened muscles and increase the range of motion of a joint.

Physiological effects result from the physical and chemical changes that occur when the body is massaged. These may include the removal of metabolic waste and inflammatory by-products, increase in blood flow to soft tissue, increased cellular metabolism, neurologically and chemically mediated arteriolar and capillary dilation, localized skin hyperemia, and increase in skin temperature. Enhanced mental clarity, generalized muscle relaxation and the reduction of pain occur via nervous system changes and are considered to be *Reflex* effects.

Psychological (mind-body) effects contribute to changes in the emotional and mental processes and their effect on body. Noxious stimulation of the nervous system may be reduced resulting in stress reduction, improved well-being, and relaxation. Some authors also discuss *Energetic* effects, which are due to "energy balancing".

Refer to the Anatomy, Physiology, and Pathology sections of this review for detailed information on the body systems, their functions, and pathologies.

1. Circulatory Systems - *Blood and Lymph*

The (blood) *circulatory system* delivers oxygen, nutrients, and other important components to the cells. It also removes carbon dioxide, metabolic by-products, and other substances including numerous chemical compounds which can be toxic to the body if found in sufficient quantities.

The *lymphatic system* supplements the blood circulatory system returning interstitial fluid (lymph) to the blood. This system is **not** pressurized by the heart and depends primarily on the contraction of **voluntary skeletal muscle** to move the lymph throughout the body. Lymphatic capillaries are more permeable than blood vessels and accept larger particles, the kind which result from cell breakdown. These materials, along with foreign substances (virus and bacteria), are removed, broken down or consumed by lymphocytes located throughout this system. This increase in blood and lymph circulation is the most widely recognized physiological effect of massage.

Massage facilitates the removal of metabolic waste and inflammatory by-products by the increase in blood flow and also by increased lymph formation and removal. *The delivery of oxygen and nutrients to cells is enhanced through massage because of the improved vascular and lymphatic circulation, reducing ischemia.* Local blood flow is increased by arteriolar and capillary dilation.

Studies show that massage, through compression, empties venous beds, lowers venous pressure, and increases capillary blood flow. It results in chemically mediated arteriolar and capillary dilation resulting in localized skin hyperemia and increased skin temperature, and results in changes in blood flow induced by autonomic vascular reflexes, affecting blood pressure and heart rate (initially increased and then reduced). Conventional massage may produce an increase in blood pressure and heart rate. However, *slow* stroking massage reduces heart rate and blood pressure.

Studies also show that, massage can affect a release of *histamines* and acetylcholine, which results in vasodilation and increases in blood flow. Lymph flow is increased because massage opens up blood capillaries that may be closed, increasing the total capillary surface area, and increasing venous pressure which in turn increases the capillary pressure. The net result is increased filtration and rate of lymph formation. Applying massage in a proximal direction reduces edema because of the resulting shift of edema fluid from the tissues to the blood and the accompanying removal of various chemical compounds. There is also an increase in urine volume and excretion.

2. Integumentary System

Massage may improve the condition of the skin by increasing the blood flow, resulting in a rise in skin temperature and perspiration, which facilitates sebaceous secretions.

3. Immune System

Recent studies at the University of Miami Medical School's Touch Research Institute concluded that the immune system is positively affected by massage. There was a significant increase in Natural Killer (NK) cell numbers in an HIV control group. There was also a significant decrease in anxiety and increase in relaxation. The study concluded that the decrease in anxiety was significantly correlated with the increase in NK cell number. Studies have also shown a decrease in anxiety and increased immune response among cancer patients who receive massage. In *The Stress of Life*, Hans Selye, MD., notes that the main regulators of the stress syndrome are the endocrine and nervous system. The sympathetic nervous system stimulates production of adrenaline, cortisol, and acetylcholine, necessary for the "fight or flight syndrome". However, prolonged production of these chemicals (such as long periods of stress) lower the immune system by destroying white blood cells (lymphoid and eosinophils). Massage has been shown to reduce the effects of anxiety related to stress.

4. Muscular System

Massage may promote muscle relaxation, relief of spasms and cramps, relief from muscular pain syndromes, prevention and treatment of delayed muscle soreness, improved athletic performance and enhanced recovery, rehabilitation following muscle injury, and the treatment of immobilized or paralyzed muscle. Let's take a look at the effects of massage on muscle tissue. These conditions include:

> **a.** *Muscle relaxation* is a widely accepted benefit of massage, supported by studies. However, since skeletal muscle contraction is entirely under the control of the nervous system, it must be concluded that massage affects nerve activity, which in turn causes muscle relaxation. Also, muscle tone is ultimately controlled by the brain and indirectly affected by the individual's emotional state. Over stimulation of the nervous system can result in muscle spasm and cramps. A person's psychological state has a direct impact on the *nociceptive* impulses originating from peripheral tissue. Epinephrine is released, which activates the peripheral neuoreceptors. Sympathetic activity that results from stress can aggravate the nociceptive impulses originating from the soft tissue injury. Studies support the effect massage has on the reduction of anxiety. This reduction may have a sedating effect on the over-stimulation of the nervous system, which in turn may result in muscle relaxation.

b. *Spasms and cramps* have long been treated by massage. However, there are no specific studies to support this treatment. Muscle spasm occurs to splint or prevent movement of injured tissue, and when fluid & electrolyte imbalances occur. Compression of the contracted muscle produces a reflex response in tendon *proprioceptors*, which are thought to contribute to muscle spasm relief. Massage techniques that slowly stretch the hypertonic muscle may bring about relaxation by mechanisms involving the quieting of *muscle spindle cells* by the stimulation of *Golgi Tendon Organs*. Cramps also respond to *Reciprocal Inhibition* treatment.

The muscle spindles and Golgi tendon organs are partners. The muscle spindle measures the length of a muscle's fibers and the speed with which the length is changing. When a muscle spindle is stretched beyond what is "normal" resting length, the motor neurons are excited, and the muscle contracts immediately to reset the "normal" length. The Golgi tendon organs measure the tension in connective tissue components that develops as a result of changes in muscle tonus. The Golgi tendon organ has an *inhibitory* effect on the motor neuron. When the tension exceeds "normal" the Golgi tendon organs inhibit the motor neurons, reducing the stimulation and reducing the tension back down to "normal." These mechanisms are in operation when a joint is taken through a complete range of motion, and in those manipulative techniques in which the patient resists an opposing force applied by the therapist.

c. *Hypertonic muscles* (sustained increased muscular tone) can be caused by *ischemia*. Studies support the belief that massage reduces ischemia and its harmful effects. The relaxation of the hypertonic muscle, resulting from the manipulation of tissue and the corresponding nerve reflex effects, which decrease the muscle tone, is the first and essential step in improving blood circulation, which reduces ischemia.

d. *Delayed onset muscle soreness* (pain occurring 24 to 48 hours following new types of exercise, over-exercise by inactive individuals, or accelerated training), is thought to be the result of trauma to the microscopic muscle filaments, and may be reduced by massage. Massage is believed to facilitate the recovery time through improved circulation, the removal of metabolic waste products, and the prevention of fibrosis.

e. *Myofascial pain* results from trigger points, areas of abnormal nerve activity in skeletal muscle or fascia, which are tender and refer pain. Metabolic waste products build up in these areas, chemicals excite pain nerve endings, and nutrients & oxygen are decreased. A cycle of muscle spasm and pain result. Terms such as myalgia, fibrositis, fascitis, etc. are used to describe myofascial pain. Applying deep compressive forces to the area can effectively treat trigger points. This process releases pain killing neuropeptides, stimulates pressure receptors, creating competing stimuli.

5. Nervous System

The nervous system controls all soft tissue. The muscle cell depends on its motor neuron to initiate contractions, relaxation, and determine its resting length. The muscle cell's health is dependent on the constant electrical energy received from the nerve. If the muscle doesn't receive this electrical energy, it will begin to atrophy. Noxious irritation of tissue causes nociceptive responses, which result in the symptom of pain. This information is ultimately transmitted to the brain by the peripheral nerves and spinal cord. According to John Yates, Ph.D., *A Physician's Guide to Therapeutic Massage,* there are three ways massage may reduce pain. It may act ***directly on the source*** of the pain to alleviate nociceptive stimulation (reducing ischemia), it may ***act centrally*** to alter the processing of nociceptive input (trigger point therapy or friction), or it may affect the ***conduction*** of pain impulses in the peripheral nerves (ice massage).

Chemicals, such as enkephalins, serotonin, and endorphins, inhibit neurostimulators. When the body is touched, the pain control system of the brain and spinal cord may be activated, releasing these chemicals. Trigger point therapy stimulates proprioceptive nerve endings, helping with enkephalin release and interrupting the pain-contraction cycle.

The "Gate Theory" states that the brain allows certain impulses to override others. When a secondary stimulation comes into the cord, it overrides the reflex arc, which is stimulating the pain signals. These over-riding stimuli include heat, cold, acupuncture, pressure, and friction. Studies conclude that deep friction massage in the treatment of tendonous and ligamentous injuries produce an analgesic effect, which can be explained by the Gate Theory. Ice massage has proven to effectively block nerve conduction and produce an analgesic affect. Another term used to describe this phenomenon is "hyperstimulation analgesia."

6. Respiratory System

Chronic lung disease causes certain musculoskeletal changes when the accessory muscles become involved in helping the patient breathe (i.e., decreased rib-cage mobility and stiff neck). The patient is anxious and tense due to these changes. Massage may produce relaxation through a temporary reduction in anxiety and tension. Chest percussion, in combination with postural drainage, is also used for certain congestive respiratory disorders (CF, & Bronchiectasis).

E. Massage Strokes

There are five basic massage strokes: *Gliding (effleurage), Kneading (petrissage), Tapotement, Friction,* and *Vibration.* Each stroke has a definite purpose. The *pressure* should be adjusted to the body part being massaged (lighter pressure over bony areas). Massage strokes begin with light pressure and increase slowly; always communicating with the client to insure *pressure* (thrust) does not exceed the client's tolerance (*using verbal & visual feedback*), and is appropriate for the body area and condition. The pressure strokes should follow the venous flow (**centripetal**), and pressure is reduced on the return stroke. The strokes used should be geared to meet the objective of the massage.

1. **Gliding** *(effleurage)* - Any stroke that glides over the skin without attempting to move the deep muscle mass. This is the *most widely used massage stroke*. The therapist's hands are molded to the body, fingers together, hands relaxed, wrists in alignment, using firm even pressure. Basic effleurage may be performed with the palms and fingers, the thumbs, fists, or forearms. *Shingles* effleurage refers to alternate stroking, with strokes overlapping each other and one hand always in contact with the receiver. *Nerve Strokes* are very light movements performed with the fingertips gently brushing the skin (or sheet) and are often used to complete a relaxing massage. *Mennel's* superficial stroking is very light effleurage performed on a limb, moving in only one direction. The return stroke is through the air just above the skin surface. Effleurage strokes are rhythmical, and the speed of movement should be constant.

The **purpose** of gliding strokes is to:
   a. Begin and end the massage
   b. Spread the lubricant.
   c. Accustom the client to your touch.
   d. Evaluate the client's soft tissue.
   e. Determine client's pain tolerance (less invasive).
   f. Relax the client (long strokes from head to coccyx).
   g. Stimulate (very light gliding strokes - feathering).
   h. Stretch muscle tissue (deep, gliding strokes following the direction of the muscle fiber).
   i. Broaden muscle tissue (deep, gliding movements transverse to muscle fiber).
   j. Enhance venous blood and lymphatic flow (reduce certain types of edema and improve circulation).

2. **Kneading** *(Petrissage)* - Manipulation of the fleshy areas (muscle belly) using a technique which lifts, grasps, rolls, and compresses the muscle mass. The therapist can use two fingers or one hand on small areas and both hands on larger areas. The pressure is firm. Pressure strokes move forcefully centripetally and glide back with less pressure. Arms and shoulders are relaxed with elbows close to the body. *Skin rolling* and *Fulling* are variation of the kneading technique. In *skin rolling*, the fingers are used to alternately pick up and pull the skin away from the underlying tissues as the thumbs glide along in the direction of movement. No lubricant is used in skin rolling. *Fulling* involves the gentle lifting and spreading of superficial tissue, as if to make more space between the soft tissue components. Fulling is typically administered using both hands to pick up, separate, and stretch the soft tissues. Compression is also considered a form of petrissage and may be applied with the thumbs, palms, or fists. *Ischemic* (static) *compression* causes blanching / reflex vasodilation to increase local circulation.

The **purpose** of kneading is to:
   a. Assist venous return and removal of metabolic by-products.
   b. Free adhesions in the muscle belly.
   c. Enhance fluid movement in deeper tissue.
   d. Stretch muscle tissue.
   e. Stretch fascia (skin rolling).

3. Friction uses various techniques to reach the deeper tissue, especially around joint spaces and bony prominances (tendons, ligaments, and their attachments). Friction requires direct pressure on the skin with *no* gliding to affect the underlying structures. These movements permit the therapist to penetrate the deeper tissue *gradually*. Release of the tissue should also be gradual. Therapists should keep their joints in alignment. The pressure comes from the therapist's *body*, not just the thumbs or fingers. Friction may include small *Circular* movements that move the tissue *under* the skin, *Cyriax's* cross-fiber or transverse friction is applied perpendicular to long axis of muscle (the preferred treatment for fibrous tissue injuries), *Storm's* parallel strokes and palmar friction are compressive movements which are rhythmical and pumping in nature and commonly used in fleshy or muscular areas (i.e. gluteals in sports massage). Linear Friction is also known as *Chucking*. Specifically, *"chucking"* is described as a series of quick movements in which the therapist firmly grasps the soft tissues and moves them proximally and distally along the axis of an extremity. Rolling, wringing, and shaking are variations of friction commonly applied to the extremities.

The **purpose** of friction is to:
   a. Separate tissue and break down adhesions.
   b. Increase circulation.
   c. Soften deposits between fascia.
   d. Aid absorption of fluid around joints

4. Tapotement *(percussive movements)* includes techniques that strike, tap, beat, and slap, and are highly stimulating. These movements should be rapid and alternating. Descriptive terms used are *quacking, hacking, cupping, slapping, squishing, tapping, pincement,* and *beating*. These movements do not have much force, and the therapist's wrists remain relaxed. These movements are not often used but have a definite purpose and should be used when appropriate. They should not be used over the *kidneys*, abnormally contracted muscles, and any sensitive areas.

The **purpose** of tapotement is to:
   a. Stimulate (as in athletic events).
   b. Increase circulation (amputee's stump w/ 70% alcohol).
   c. Loosen phlegm (respiratory conditions).
   d. Tone muscle.

5. Vibration is a continuous oscillating, quivering, shaking, or trembling movement made by the therapist's hand (or electrical device) being placed firmly against a body part. The therapist's wrist and fingers are stable, and the movement comes through the forearm, wrist, and fingers, not just the hand. Vibration may be fine (as applied to a small area with the fingertips), coarse (and involve shaking a large muscle), or used over a nerve root, trunk, or branch.

The **purpose** of vibration is to:
   a. Soothe and relax (light vibration).
   b. Desensitize an area or point.
   c. Stimulate when applied with pressure.

(**Passive Touch** was included as an additional stroke by J.H. Kellogg, and is further described by Tappan as "skilled touch with intention.")

F. Joint Movements

The Range of Motion is the natural movement of a joint from one extreme of its articulation to the other. All joints have some normal restriction, such as bone to bone and the tension of ligaments and muscles. Ideally, every joint should be able to move through its complete range of motion (ROM) without discomfort. (See ROM Chart in Kinesiology & Biomechanics section) If the muscles, tendons and connective tissue surrounding a joint are taken through their full ROM on a regular basis, abnormal restrictions do not occur. Abnormal restrictions are caused by tense muscles, injured tissues, inflammation, aging, muscle imbalance (i.e. result of weight training or repetitive use of the flexors), inactivity, overuse while not maintaining full ROM, or other pathological conditions, resulting in pain when the joint attempts to go through its full ROM. Therapists use joint movements to assess and treat loss of ROM. Joint movements are used to help restore mobility or increase flexibility of a joint. The body part involved should be *properly supported and the joint isolated*. Assessment and treatment methods include:

1. Passive joint movements - Therapist stretches & moves the body part, with client remaining relaxed.

Assessment through passive joint movement provides information about the health of associated soft tissue structures – normal joint motion should not produce pain or crepitus.

The amount and quality of joint motion are commonly described as being either normal, primary motion (that which would be accomplished through normal active movement), or accessory motion (that which is still within normal physiological limits yet, can only be demonstrated by assisted movement). These qualities and limits of movement are often described as "end feel." Each type of "end feel" describes the nature of joint function found at the end of that particular joint's range of motion. The following are common descriptions:

a. *Hard end feel* (bone to bone end feel) results when the boney components of a joint contact each other at the end of the joint range of motion.

b. *Soft end feel* (soft tissue approximation) results when the soft tissue components (muscle) of structures surrounding a joint contact and compress each other near the end of the joint range of motion. (the contact of the biceps muscle with the forearm during flexion of the elbow).

c. *Tissue stretch* (springy end feel) results when the soft tissue components of a joint limit further motion at the end of the joint range of motion. This type of end feel is also described as being "leathery" in nature, as the ligaments and joint capsule tissues exhibit a leather-like stretch before halting movement.

d. *Muscle spasms* tend to limit joint motion by abruptly and prematurely halting motion before reaching normal physiological limits. Pain is often produced when spasms limit ROM.

e. *Springy block* is a pathological end feel associated with a loose component of the joint moving among the other joint components. An example would be found where loose pieces of meniscus move throughout the joint capsule and disrupt normal motion. Pain may or may not be produced.

f. *Empty end feel* occurs when pain limits joint motion where no physiological or mechanical barriers exist.

2. **Active joint movements** - Client participates by contracting the muscles involved in the movement.

3. **Active Assisted joint movements** - Client performs a motion with the assistance of the therapist.

G. Stretching

Exercises and movements aimed at lengthening and strengthening the muscle, and taking the joint through its full ROM may improve flexibility and mobility, improving the quality of life that has been affected by restrictions in movement and accompanying pain. Breathing should be slow and rhythmical. The client should breathe slowly while holding the stretch, inhale as body returns to starting point, and exhale when muscle is being stretched. Isolate the muscle to be stretched. The stretch should be taken to the point of *mild tension* where the client can maintain *relaxation of the muscle being stretched.* Overstretching is counter productive. The stretch reflex (a nerve reflex) will signal the muscle to contract when stretched too far.

The **purpose** of stretching is to:
1. Increase and maintain complete ROM.
2. Relieve muscle and joint soreness.
3. Improve mobility/movement.
4. Lengthen fascia and improve elasticity.
5. Prevent re-injury and strengthen tissue.
6. (Pre-activity) - Increase tissue temperature by increased metabolic rate.
7. (Post-activity) - Increase blood flow to area (bringing nutrients to area and removing metabolic and inflammatory by-products).

Types of stretching include:

1. Static (assisted) - Therapist gently stretches the muscle until resistance is met & holds until the muscle releases (usually 10-20 seconds). Static stretching stimulates Golgi tendon organs and thus inhibits motor neuron activity.

2. Static (unassisted) - Stretching procedure in which muscle is stretched and held in stretched position for a specified period of time. This technique is performed by the client applying a small torque to a muscle after it is positioned at its end ROM. Yoga is an example. Yoga is a form of stretching, utilizing specific *postures*, *breathing techniques* and practices, which include *balancing the chakras* (energy centers of the body).

3. Proprioceptive Neuromuscular Facilitation technique (assisted) - In PNF, the body part is moved to the point where tension is experienced. This position is held for 10 seconds, the individual then contracts the muscle against resistance for 5 seconds, and then the body part is further stretched gently until tension is experienced again. The procedure is repeated 3 or 4 times until the desired increase in flexibility is obtained. This method is also known as contract-relax or **post-isometric relaxation** technique. (Following an isometric contraction, there is an immediate period in which motor neuron impulses are inhibited).

4. Ballistic - Bobbing or bouncing forces used with body momentum. This is **not recommended** because it can aggravate the muscle by creating small muscle tears and may initiate the stretch reflex, causing rapid contraction of muscle via stimulation of muscle spindle cells.

5. Passive - Slow, steady movement using gentle force to lengthen tissue, but is obtained only when all voluntary and reflex muscular resistance is eliminated.

6. Reciprocal Inhibition - Contract antagonist to muscle being stretched. This technique allows for relaxation of muscle being stretched because it will be inhibited and thus relax when antagonist is contracted. This technique may be useful for **muscle cramping**. (ex: contract quadriceps if hamstrings are cramping)

H. Indications and Precautions for Massage

Massage has something to offer almost everyone. However, the treatment should be tailored to each individual's condition. Therapists must be alert to *undiagnosed* conditions. If a client's pain **persists**, refer to the appropriate health care professional. Certain conditions warrant precautions. Research, and when in doubt, it is best to exercise caution and check with the physician prior to the massage. The following pages list some indicated diseases/disorders *with any accompanying precautions.* (**SUBACUTE** phase only).

Condition	Indications (Precautions)
Acne/psoriasis/dermatitis	Non-contagious, but *avoid* affected area.
Alzheimer's Disease	May *reduce muscular spasm* & *increase* psychological *well-being.* Obtain Dr.'s O.K.
Amputations	Precaution: broken skin - may *improve circulation*.
Amyotrophic lateral sclerosis (Lou Gherig's Disease)	May *reduce muscle spasm* and *increase* psychological *well-being*. Obtain Dr.'s O.K.
Angina pectoris (Other heart disorders: myocardial infarction and hypertensive heart disease)	May *vasodilate and relax*, but *precautions*. Check with physician before massaging. Massage *slow & easy, avoid all* chronic ischemic heart *endangerment sites, avoid abdominal massage* because possibility of increasing the pressure on the inferior vena cava and overworking heart. A*void massaging in prone or left side-lying positions,* which tend to return excessive amounts of blood to the heart & overwork heart. Advise client to sit up and get off table slowly.
Arteriosclerosis	*Precaution*: Carotid artery - plaque may break loose; could be associated thrombi, aneurysms, etc. *Local massage should be avoided.* Check with physician.
Arthritis	*Rheumatoid* - Avoid affected joint(s) in acute inflammatory stage. Paraffin bath recommended. *Osteoarthritis - avoid friction of involved joints*; *range of motion is indicated*; be aware of possible bone spurs & avoid area.
Asthma	May *reduce the stress* component & loosen intercostals.

Condition	Indications (Precautions)
Bells Palsy	May help *reduce related anxiety*.
Benign Tumor	Avoid *immediate area* because massage may break its capsule.
Bronchitis (chronic)	Check with physician. May *reduce* thoracic and chest *muscular spasms* but use *caution* because it can be an *infectious disease.*
Burns	Precaution: Check with physician; if completely healed, may help reduce scare tissue.
Bursitis	Precaution: Avoid deep work over affected area; may increase circulation & assist with removal of inflammatory by-products.
Cancer	*Precaution:* Massage may aid in the metastasis of the disease; obtain physician's OK. *Subtle energy techniques* may be appropriate and can *reduce the anxiety & related stress.*
Carpal Tunnel Syndrome	May improve circulation and relax muscles involved.
Cerebral Palsy	Motor disorder - *Obtain physician's OK* because it is a neurological disorder affecting muscle control.
Cirrhosis	*Abdominal massage* should be *avoided*; massage of lower extremities may relieve associated edema; obtain physician's O.K. because of other problems that can result from liver damage.
Constipation	*Precaution: pregnancy* - Abdominal massage may assist with movement or disrupt blockage.
Contractures	May slow down contraction or help prevent.
Contusions (Bruise - non-acute)	*Precaution: bleeding*; Avoid affected area; may improve circulation.
Cystic fibrosis	Check with physician. *Local* massage may be *contraindicated* in the *area of the pancreas* if inflamed; *tapotement* may help ease blockage of the lungs.

Condition	Indications (Precautions)
Decubitis Ulcers	Usually a *preventive* measure; may increase circulation to area. ***Do not massage affected area***.
Degenerative Disc Disease	*May help prevent contractures*; ***Obtain physician's OK***. Relaxation may disrupt guarding of injured area.
Diabetes Mellitus	*Precautions* necessary due to progression of of disease such as neuropathy, metabolic, and vascular complications (i.e. atherosclerosis, decreased sensory ability & kidney problems). - ***Obtain physician's OK.***
Digestive problem	***Precaution: pregnancy*** -Abdominal massage can *facilitate peristalsis*.
Dysmenorrhea	Pain may be reduced by decreasing circulatory congestion.
Dislocation	***Obtain Dr.'s OK***. Do not massage directly on the joint until swelling is reduced & pain level permits. *Stretching* may begin when ligament damage is sufficiently healed.
Edema	If caused by inactivity or post operative procedures - *may improve blood and lymph circulation* & reduce swelling. ***Determine cause: Check with Dr.***
Emphysema	May reduce anxiety/relax muscles involved with breathing.
Endometrial Hyperplasia (Endometriosis, Endometritis)	***Precaution:*** *Local* massage on *lower abdomen* should be avoided.
Fibromyalgia, Fibrosis, Fibrositis & Fibromyositis	Kneading, passive movement, & deep friction may loosen adhesions, prevent further formation, & reduce associated stress *(often hypersensitive to touch)*.
Fractures	While in cast, work above site to reduce edema & below to improve circulation. After caste is off, gradually work toward the injured site, but not on the site ***until Dr. OK's*** & ensures there is complete union. Passive/active/resistive exercises stretch atrophied muscles.

Condition	Indications (Precautions)
Headaches (tension)	Reduce tension/relaxation of affected muscles. (also for cervicogenic / trigger point HA)
Herniated Disc	*Precaution: Avoid area; **Obtain physician's OK.***
Hypertension	*Determine cause, **Obtain physician's OK.*** – May reduce high blood pressure caused by anxiety. If extreme, do not massage because increased chance of thrombus formation.
Injured limb (non-acute)	Massage proximal to injury first. May improve circulation.
Insomnia	Long, light-gliding strokes from occiput to coccyx may be relaxing.
Laminectomy	*Precaution: Avoid immediate area; **Obtain Dr.'s OK.***
Lipoma, Sebaceous Cyst	Recognize; massage not contraindicated. Make referral to health care professional for treatment.
Mental conditions	*Precaution: Medications may affect sensitivity to pain; **Obtain physician's OK.*** May aggravate some conditions, such as manic depressant.
Multiple Sclerosis	Demyelination / neurological symptoms - *Precaution: compromised sensitivity.* May help muscle spasm & increase psychological well-being.
Muscle cramps	Short, gliding strokes from tendon to muscle belly may cause a reflexive relaxation of the muscle. (Reciprocal Inhibition stretching technique may relax).
Neuralgia	May help alleviate pain through reduction in anxiety and release of endorphins.
Neurasthenia	May reduce anxiety related to chronic fatigue syndrome
Nonunion fractures	*Precaution: avoid immediate area.*
Parkinson's Disease	Neurological disorder - ***Obtain physician's OK.*** May help muscle spasm & psychological well-being.

Condition	Indications (Precautions)
Peripheral Neuritis	Light vibration is effective - *Other forms of massage may aggravate condition.*
Poliomyelitis	May increase circulation to paralyzed area.
Postural Deviations	Scoliosis, kyphosis, lordosis - May relax muscles affected.
Pregnancy	Precaution: Avoid abdominal massage during first trimester.
Psoriasis, Urticaria	*Noncontagious dermatitis* - massage nonaffected area; may reduce stress which can aggravate condition.
Raynaud's Disease	May increase circulation & relax contracted muscles.
Scar tissue	*Precaution: Avoid massage for 6-8 weeks* after surgery; cross fiber friction may disrupt/help reduce formation.
Sciatica	May help reduce anxiety; **Obtain Dr.'s O.K.**
Sprains	*R.I.C.E.* first 48-72 hours; massage may speed recovery through improved circulation.
Strains	Same as Sprains.
Subluxation	**Obtain Dr.'s OK**. If no inflammation, can reduce muscle spasm.
Tendonitis	Deep friction preferred treatment-May disrupt lesions and produce temporary analgesia.
Tenosynovitis	Same as Tendonitis.
Thoracic Outlet Syndrome	Precaution: Working near brachial plexus. May relax contracted muscles and reduce nerve compression/ entrapment.

Condition	Indications (Precautions)
TMJ dysfunction	May relax muscles and help relieve symptoms. *Check with dentist* to make sure massage will not interfere with dental procedures, etc.
Trigeminal neuralgia	(Tic Douloreux) - May relax spasms & produce temporary neuralgia.
Torticollis	May relax affected muscles & relieve anxiety. *Obtain Dr.'s OK.*
Tuberculosis	Debilitative & infectious; *Obtain physician's OK.*
Whiplash (post acute)	May relax muscles & relieve symptoms. *Obtain Dr.'s OK.*

I. Contraindications for Massage

Certain conditions warrant special consideration and massage may not be appropriate at all. Some disorders would be contraindicated for Swedish or deep tissue massage but may benefit from polarity therapy, therapeutic touch, and other subtle energy techniques. *Always check with the physician.* Contraindications include:

Condition	Contraindication
Abdominal Aneurysm	Massage of *abdomen contraindicated.*
Abnormal lumps	*Avoid the immediate area* & *diplomatically* suggest the client see a physician to determine cause of lump.
Abnormal Sensation (diabetes, stroke, some medications, Hyperesthesia, & certain neurological disorders)	*Be cautious* & *obtain physician's OK.* Research condition.
Anemia (hemolytic)	*Mechanical pressure* on surface vessels could *cause more harm.*
Atherosclerosis	*Avoid endangerment sites:* posterior tibial, popliteal, femoral artery, axillary, brachial, radial, carotid, & temporal artery. General massage contraindicated if severe because movement of fluids could cause embolism.

Condition	Contraindication
Bleeding (ecchymosis, hematomas, etc.)	*Avoid* area.
Bone Fractures	*Avoid immediate area* unless physician OKs massage.
Bursitis	Acute bursitis; can increase *inflammatory* response.
Carcinoma (basal/squamous cell)	***Obtain physician's OK.*** Massage may aid in the metastasis of disease; energy work may benefit stress/anxiety reduction.
Circulatory System Disorders: (certain hypertension, cardiac decompensation, & cardiac arrhythmias)	***Research*** carefully & ***obtain physician's O.K.***
Compromised Immune System (AIDS)	Use ***Universal precautions,*** hygiene, & obtain physician's O.K.
Edema	*Understand cause*; edema due to heart decompensation, infections, kidney ailments, or obstructions are contraindicated.
Elderly clients (Atherosclerosis is common condition)	May *bruise* easily; pressure should be adjusted accordingly. (Do not do deep massage unless physician orders.) Avoid extreme neck rotation & the carotid artery area; plaque could break loose.
Extreme Fatigue	Recent & undiagnosed *extreme* fatigue may be indicator of many serious conditions (such as cancer, auto-immune disease, chronic infection, etc). Exercise caution & make appropriate referral to health care professional.
Fever (acute)	Massage not desired; indication of problem & often indicator of infection.
Hernia	*Avoid* massage on or near *affected area*.

Condition	Contraindication
Impetigo, warts, ringworm, scabies, & other infectious skin conditions (i.e. bacterial, viral, fungal, & parasitic)	*Contagious* - Do not massage.
Infectious diseases (cold, flu, Reye's syndrome, tuberculosis, arthritis, etc.)	May *intensify* the condition & possibly spread the infection and/or *expose* the therapist.
Inflammation -*Acute*: (cellulitis, pyelitis, Crohn's disease, cystitis, diverticulitis, encephalitis, hepatitis, Lyme Disease, lymphangitis, osteomyelitis, pancreatitis, peritonitis, phlebitis, sinusitis, Systemic Lupus, thrombophlebitis, urethritis, & *areas* of *redness/pain/heat/swelling*)	*Avoid* local area of inflammation; *Obtain Dr.'s OK* for general massage
Loss of Integrity (recent surgeries & accompanying scar tissue formation, chronic sacroiliac joint subluxation, severe rheumatoid arthritis)	*Research & obtain physician's OK.*
Malignant melanomas (undiagnosed skin conditions)	Can *metastasize.* Avoid immediate area & *obtain physicians O.K.* before any massage.
Medications (muscle relaxants/immunosuppressants/ blood thinners)	*Understand* what they *do*; *check with physician.*
Migraine Headache	*Caution during attacks; obtain Dr.'s OK.* Pressure-point massage may be helpful.
Open sores/lacerations, etc.	*Avoid* area.
Osteoporosis	Bone is deteriorating; can break. *Obtain physician's OK.*
Osteomalacia (rickets), Osteitis, Fibrosa Cystica, Osteitis deformans (Paget's disease)	*Contraindicated* due to fragile condition of the bone, muscle weakness and side effects of drugs used.

Condition	Contraindication
Severe muscle injury	Avoid deep massage for 5-7 days; *R.I.C.E.*
Substance abuse	*Do no treat client while under the influence* of drugs and alcohol. Reschedule & explain that you will not massage if they are in this condition.
Unexplained Pain	Question client to determine *cause* before proceeding; may need to reschedule & advise client to see appropriate health care professional.
Varicose Veins	*Do not* massage *distal* to area or directly to affected area. However, massage *is not contraindicated proximal* to the area and can be helpful.

J. Endangerment Sites

Certain areas of the body warrant **special precautions and considerations** because of the **underlying anatomical structures**. Massage techniques could injure these structures. In most of these areas major nerves, vessels, arteries, or organs are exposed. The charts list endangerment sites, location, and structures involved.

Endangerment Site	Location	Structure Involved
Abdomen	Upper area under ribs	*Right Side:* Liver & Gall Bladder *Left Side:* Spleen *Deep Center:* Aorta
Anterior Triangle of Neck	Bordered by: Mandible, SCM, & Trachea	Carotid Artery; Int. Jugular Vein; Vagus Nerve & Lymph Nodes
Axilla	Armpit	Axillary, Median, Ulnar & Musculocutaneous Nerves; Axillary Artery & Lymph Nodes
Cubital area of Elbow	Anterior bend of elbow	Median Nerve; Radial & Ulnar Arteries; Median Cubital Vein

Endangerment Site	Location	Structure Involved
Femoral Triangle	Bordered by: Sartorius, Adductor Longus, & Inguinal Ligament	Femoral Nerve; Artery & Vein; Great Saphenous Vein & Lymph Nodes
Inferior to Ear	Notch posterior to ramus of Mandible	External carotid artery; styloid process, Facial nerve
Medial Brachium	Upper, inner arm Between Biceps & Triceps	Ulnar, Median, & Musculocutaneous Nerves; Brachial Artery; Basilic Vein & Lymph Nodes
Popliteal Fossa	Posterior knee Bordered by Gastroc/ Hamstrings	Tibial nerve; Popliteal Artery & Vein
Posterior Triangle of Neck	Bordered by: SCM, Trapezius, Clavicle	Brachial Plexus; Subclavian Artery; Brachiocephelic & External Jugular Veins; Lymph Nodes
Ulnar Notch of Elbow	Funny Bone	Ulnar Nerve
Upper Lumbar Area	Inferior to ribs/lateral to spine	**Kidneys** (avoid percussion)

K. Professional Image

Personal appearance should be neat and clean. Dress should be comfortable (to allow freedom of movement), but professional and appropriate for place of business. Confidence and trust should be communicated. Because of the close contact between the therapist and client, your attitude and touch should one of understanding, but never personal.

L. Hygiene

Personal hygiene: first and foremost **clean hands/nails** (nails clipped), good oral hygiene and unscented deodorant (many people are allergic to perfumes). **Universal Precautions** should be used when appropriate to protect the therapist and client.

M. Posture & Body Mechanics

Poor posture and body mechanics can result in fatigue and muscle strain. Good body mechanics result in safe and efficient movement, which increase the strength and power available to the therapist and reduce the possibility of injury. Proper body mechanics enhance the quality and effectiveness of the massage. Body weight should be *evenly* distributed on both feet, keeping the body in proper alignment. When necessary, weight should shift from one foot to the other. Movement should originate from the *"Tan Tien"* or center of gravity, which is located just anterior to the 4th Lumbar vertebra. The main source of strength comes from the lower body, not the arms and shoulders. The therapist should use their entire body weight and lean into the movement.

Properly *balanced* on both feet with knees flexed, the therapist's legs, pelvis, and torso provide the leverage and strength needed to apply pressure. ***Do not bend at the waist-- Bend the knees and keep the back straight.*** Hands and elbows should remain close to the body, and shoulders and wrists should remain ***relaxed***, conserving the therapist's energy. The elbow, forearm, fists, and pressure bars provide useful substitutes for the hand and fingers on certain body parts, giving needed relief when necessary.

Also, the massage table height is important. Adjust the height to allow for correct posture, for the technique to be used and the client's size. The ***Archer Stance*** is most commonly used and involves the practitioner taking a position with shoulders at an angle to the massage table, one-foot forward and pointing in the direction of the movement. Alternately, the ***Horse Stance*** is described as having both feet and the shoulders perpendicular to the edge of the massage table.

Proper care of the therapist's hands and wrists is necessary to prevent injury and disease (arthritis, carpal tunnel syndrome, tendonitis, etc.). Keeping wrists in alignment and thumbs straight, along with flexibility and strengthening exercises provide a good preventive routine. Avoiding small repetitive movements with your wrists, fingers, and thumbs can help avoid carpal tunnel syndrome. When injury does occur, immediate rest is necessary. Massage should ***not*** be resumed until the injury is healed. More serious damage may result if you continue.

Practices for maintaining strength, balance, and body control include the following techniques: ***Centering***, which is accomplished by concentrating on the body's physical center of gravity (tan tien) and by learning self-assurance. ***Grounding***, which involves visualization and controlled breathing to negate negative influences of the recipient, oneself or the surroundings. ***Grinding Corn***, an exercise to develop good posture and balance that involves standing with feet apart, bending knees and moving the hands together in a large flat oval. The ***Wheel,*** which teaches deep breathing, posture and moving from tan tien by shifting body weight from one foot to the other while tracing large vertical circles with the hands in front of the body and rhythmic breathing. The ***Tree*** involves standing alternately on each forefoot with arms forward (as if around a tree) and deep rhythmic breathing exercises to develop strength and concentration.

N. Client Consultation

The initial interview (clear and tactful communication) and the client intake form are extremely important. They are the therapist's primary tools to ensure that the client's needs are met. Guidelines are:

1. **Greeting** should be professional and friendly. (good eye contact / handshake)

2. **Introductions**: Determine who client is, why they want a massage, and explain your professional services and fee.

3. **Client intake form**: This is *essential* in determining medical history and any *pre-cautions or contraindications*. Tactfully question the client further if clarification is needed. Careful notes also help you assess and develop a treatment plan. Documentation is important because your files may be used for insurance cases or in malpractice litigation. If a client refuses to complete the form, make sure all necessary questions are answered before proceeding with the massage. If client's present health (fever, infectious disease, acute injury) or emotional states are contraindicated, do *not* proceed with the massage. Tactfully explain reasons and request they see appropriate health care provider and reschedule.

4. **Explain massage procedure**--clear instructions regarding draping and disrobing are required and can ease the client's concerns.

O. Preparing the Client for Massage

The client's comfort is critical to the success of the treatment. Make sure the room temperature (75°), lighting, and surroundings are comfortable. Explain the following:

1. The use and location of facilities.
2. Disrobing and dressing procedures.
3. Types of draping and related procedures.
4. Proper way to get on and off table and positioning.
5. The use of bolsters or pillows (necessary to insure the client's comfort and proper support).
6. The purpose and choice of lubricant (reduces friction) whether to leave on, methods of removal, and determine if client is allergic to oils or cream.

Draping Methods: 1) ***Diaper Draping***, also known as *Contoured Draping* - uses one or two towels to drape genitals (males & females), breasts (females), and a table cover (sheet or large towel). This is suitable for warm rooms. 2) ***Top Cover Draping***, also known as *Flat Draping* - uses a table cover and one large towel or sheet to cover the entire body. 3) ***Full Sheet Draping*** - uses one full size (at least a double, minimum 80" wide) sheet to cover the table and to wrap the client. 4) ***Tenting*** - Technique that allows client to turn over (and away from therapist) without becoming entangled in the sheet.

P. Massage Equipment

A number of factors influence equipment choices. Treatment room size (minimum 10'x12'), organization, setting, and personal business plans are major considerations.

    1. The **massage table** usually represents the largest equipment investment made. Considerations include type (stationary or portable), width, height, length, frame material, padding, weight (if portable), and fabric. Accessories for the table include face cradle, arm rest, footrest, carrying case, table skate or cart, bolsters & supportive devices. *Stationary* massage tables are more expensive, heavier and generally more stable than portable tables. They may also include the added features of easy height adjustment, storage compartments and tilting sections. *Portable* massage tables are by far the most common. Table *widths* range between 28 and 31 inches. Generally speaking, shorter therapists find it more comfortable to work across narrower tables. Large clients may need wider tables, but add-on armrests can compensate. Table *height* is a matter of the therapist's height, massage style, work environment, and personal preference. For Swedish massage, the appropriate table height should be at about the level of the therapist's knuckles or palm when standing with the arm and shoulder relaxed. For modalities requiring deeper pressure, the table may be lower to take advantage of body weight and leverage. Portable tables have an adjustable height range 22 to34 inches via variable leg height holes. Most tables are 72 or 73 inches in *length*. Face cradles add an additional 12 inches of length and accommodate nearly every client. The most common *frame materials* are wood and aluminum. Either will serve you, if it is well manufactured and maintained. The table should be able to support the weight of both the client and therapist. Foam is the common *padding* material, usually ranging from 1 and 1/2 to 3 inches in thickness. Foam density and layering influence the comfort qualities of a table. High quality tables may use more dense type foam to help resist the therapist's downward force. Table *weight* becomes an issue when the therapist travels to make home or office visits. Table *fabric* is usually some version of vinyl. A number of proprietary names are used to describe various vinyl textures and styles. Vinyl coverings are sensitive to temperature, oils, solvents, friction, ultraviolet light and sharp objects. Face cradles are either fixed or adjustable. Adjustments should be simple, quiet, and easy to make. Arm and foot rests make a table functionally larger. They should be secure and safe. Carrying cases and table skates facilitate movement and protect the table. Bolsters and supportive devices are necessary for the client's comfort and the therapist's ergonomics. Neck, ankle, and knee bolsters in 6x27 & 8x27 inch sizes are the most common. One flat side makes the bolster more stable.

    2. Lubricants are necessary to reduce friction between the therapist's hands and the client's skin. Some authors discuss the ability of a lubricant to "nourish" the client's skin, although little research exists to support this concept. The type of lubricant used is however very important. The reaction of the clients skin (and the therapist hands) to the lubricant is a very important consideration. Scented lubricants may present problems for some clients. Be sure to ask about respiratory and skin sensitivities before using any product. Hypoallergenic products are available. The capacity of the lubricant to stain linens and clothing is also an issue. Use a lubricant dispenser that does not "contaminate" the contents of the container. Pumps and tubes with holsters are available. Common lubricants include *oils, lotions, creams, cocoa butter, and powders*. Each type of lubricant has value when used appropriately. Nut and seed oils are the most common, with each having distinct qualities (viscosity, scent, shelf-life). Natural nut, seed and vegetable oils can oxidize (become rancid) easily. Protecting them from light, heat and oxygen may prolong their shelf life. Some therapists add Vitamin E to their oils and lotions to protect against oxidation. Mineral oil is generally *not recommended*. Lotions are semi-liquids, usually contain water, oils, emulsifiers, & solvents, and generally have more "drag" than pure oils, thus providing more friction. Creams are denser and more viscous than lotions, providing even more "drag". They contain less water and solvents, but otherwise are quite similar in composition to lotions. Cocoa butter provides precise control of application and significant friction for deep tissue therapy. It is the hardened fat derived from the ripe cocoa seeds of the Theobroma cacao plant. Jojoba oil (which is actually not an oil, but a liquid wax) is occasionally employed as a lubricant. Most oils, lotions and creams have the potential to stain. Various types of powders are also used in massage. Baby powder and talcum powder contain "talc" (aluminum silicate) which can cause respiratory disease when inhaled. Cornstarch will serve as a useful dry lubricant when oils, lotions, and creams are not appropriate.

Several rules should apply regardless of the lubricant used:
- a. Discuss the type of lubricant to be used with the client before beginning the massage. Rule out possible allergic reactions.
- b. Discuss how or if the lubricant will be removed following the massage. Dry towels, hot moist towels, or alcohol work well. Note that alcohol does remove moisture from the skin.
- c. Lubricant should be applied to the therapist's hands, not directly to the client. This pre-warms the lubricant and allows for dispensing the proper amount needed for a specific body area.
- d. Use the least amount necessary for the proper "glide". Additional amounts can always be used.
- e. Use little or no lubricant on the clients face. Some therapists begin a massage with the face before they handle any lubricant.
- f. Protect the client's hair from lubricant with a towel or shower cap.

3. Miscellaneous equipment may include T-Bars, stones and other devices designed to deliver precise pressure and to spare the therapist hands. Mechanical vibrators may have value in certain practices. Major types of vibrators include the orbital, oscillating and percussive. Other necessary equipment includes a sufficient supply of towels, linens, blankets, antimicrobial handsoap and gloves. Additional massage equipment may include disposable tissues, a clock, and music. Living plants add a nice touch to an office, but have the potential of eliciting an allergic response in sensitive clients.

Q. Positioning the Client

Certain muscle groups require specific positioning to enhance the treatment. Proper support should be provided through the use of pillows or bolsters. Depending on the part of the body being treated, varying positions are desirable. However, the ultimate determining factor for positioning is the **client's comfort**. Specific muscle groups and positions include:

> **l. Low back** - While lying prone, consider putting the spine into slight flexion, using a pillow under the abdomen of the client. If the client is uncomfortable lying on their abdomen, consider the side-lying position, properly supported by pillows under the cervical area and keeping the spine in alignment. When in the side-lying position, the upper arm and leg should be properly supported by pillows to ensure that the client is not assisting in maintaining this position, but completely relaxed.

> **2. Cervical and thoracic** - The client is usually lying in the prone position with the head properly supported by a face cradle. If uncomfortable, a pillow can be placed under the client's chest (may be helpful in case of Dowager's hump).

> **3. Chest** - With the client supine, a pillow under the arms will relax the pectoralis muscles.

> **4. Abdomen** - The knees should be *raised* and supported so the hip flexors and abdominal muscles are relaxed. All strokes should follow the direction of the colon as it ascends on the right, crosses, and then descends on the left. Pressure should be very gradual. Be very cautious of any ***abdominal disorders or pregnancy.***

> **5. Lower extremity** - Upper leg: when lying supine, the legs should be slightly elevated with adequate support under the knees. Lower leg: when lying prone, a pillow or bolster should be placed under the ankles, slightly elevating the lower legs. Elevating the area being massaged utilizes gravity to assist with increased venous return. The iliotibial tract (band) and tensor fasciae latae are treated more effectively when the client is in a side-lying position with proper support. Pillows should be placed between the legs to support the client's upper leg, as well as pillows providing support for the upper arm and helping to maintain proper spinal alignment and balance.

R. Sequence & Completion of Massage

Contact, once initiated, should be maintained. The sequence of massage strokes may vary, but should facilitate a smooth flow from one body part to another. The classic full body relaxation massage lasts from half to one and a half hours and includes all of the classic massage strokes, touch without movement, and passive joint movement. Oil or lotion is typically used. Beginning with the recipient in a supine or prone position is a matter of preference. The side-lying position is often used with pregnant women. For each part of the body, begin with effleurage, using lighter pressure to begin and progressing to deeper. Effleurage is typically administered in a centripetal direction (toward the heart). Follow with petrissage, using deep friction, vibration, or direct pressure for more specific work. Finish the massage with effleurage or tapotement. Very light effleurage *(Nerve Strokes)* or gentle touching without movement *(holding)* are often used to complete a relaxation massage. Recognizing and respecting the client's feedback is extremely important to the success of the massage. Client feedback can be direct or subtle: i.e., subtle feedback involves changes in **breathing patterns** and muscle **tension**; direct feedback involves therapist/client dialogue. Educate your client: explain and encourage proper breathing (breathe fully and deeply) and relaxation (visualization) techniques to enhance the massage. If a client has an emotional release, remain in contact; ask if they are O.K. and if you should continue. Be **understanding and accepting**. If your client continues to be upset, allow the client time to collect himself/herself and make a **referral** to the appropriate health care professional (psychologist, mental health counselor, etc.).

S. Specialized Massage Techniques

Various specialized techniques have evolved within the broad category of *Massage and Bodywork*. Each has a **unique focus** and **purpose**, depending on the **goal** of the therapist and client. These techniques combine various massage and bodywork practices, along with exercise and mental activities to promote healing. The following list gives a brief outline of the intent of the better-known practices:

1. **Acupressure** (Americanized Shiatsu - see Shiatsu).
   Amma/Anma - Original Korean/Japanese Therapy (see Shiatsu).

2. **Alexander Technique** - Is a contemporary form of therapy. It was developed by Fredrick Matthias Alexander (1869-1955), an actor-turned-therapist. The Alexander Technique therapist teaches or guides the student through a series of movements. In theory, poor postural patterns are replaced with simple, integrated, and healthful movements. Focus is given to gaining balance in the head-neck functional relationship. This relationship is described as "primary control". Alexander Technique International is the governing or sanctioning body.

3. **Aromatherapy** - Is an ancient science. The term "aromatherapie" was first used by the French chemist Rene Gattefosse (1881-1950). Marguerite Maury first wrote of using essential oils in massage in 1961. Aromatherapy involves the use of essential oils extracted from herbs, flowers, resin, woods, and spices. The most common method of extraction is by distillation. Other methods of extraction include hydro-diffusion, expression, enfleurage, maceration, and solvent extraction. Essential oils contain a plethora of chemical compounds or components. These components include terpenes, alcohols, phenols, aldehydes, and ketones. Each of the chemical compounds confers upon the essential oil a pharmacological property, with its own unique characteristics and therapeutic

benefits (Bergamot contains over 300 chemical compounds). Specific essential oils are blended by the aromatherapist and used in massage oils or diffusers. These oils exert their influences via two major routes. Inhaled (aromatic) oils impact olfactory receptors and enter the bloodstream by diffusion though respiratory membranes. Oils administered via massage oil (topical application) are influenced by a number of factors. These factors include the properties & amount of the oil(s) used, choice of carrier oil, and skin type and health of the client. Once topically administered, essential oils are carried by the blood to various tissues of the body where they exert their influence and are metabolized. Metabolites and unchanged chemical compounds are eliminated from the body via the lungs, kidneys, skin, and bowels. When used by a trained practitioner, the commonly used essential oils are considered to be safe. Certain essential oils carry specific cautions and contraindications. Below are listed the most popular.

Essential Oil	Indications	Contraindications
Bergamot	Anti-Anxiety, Antiseptic, Carminative	Skin Irritation, Photosensitizes
Chamomile (Roman)	Sedative, Carminative, Anti-Spasmodic	Allergic Dermatitis
Clary Sage	Calming, Menstrual Disorders	Pregnancy
Eucalyptus	Antiseptic, Bacteriostatic	Allergic Dermatitis, Toxic Internally
Geranium	Menstrual Disorders	
Lavender	Antiseptic, Muscle Pain, Calming, Sedative,	
Lemon	Antiseptic	Allergic Dermatitis
Lemongrass	Antiseptic, Calming, Sedative, Analgesic	Allergic Dermatitis
Peppermint	Stimulant, Carminative	Skin Irritation
Rosemary	Stimulant, Antiseptic	Pregnancy, Epilepsy
Sandalwood	Sedative, Antiseptic	
Tea Tree	Antiseptic, Bacteriostatic	Allergic Response
Thyme	Antiseptic, Analgesic	Hypertension
Vetiver	Calming, Anti-Anxiety	
Ylang Ylang	Sedative, Anti-Spasmodic	Skin Irritation

Carrier Oils		
Sweet Almond	Inexpensive, w/ Vitamins A, B1, B2, & E	
Avocado	Viscous, Soothing, w/ Vitamin A, & Lecithin	
Evening Primrose	Anti-inflammation, w/ GLA	
Jojoba	Emollient, Keeps well, w/ Mystiric Acid	
Olive	Viscous, w/ Monsaturated FA	
Wheatgerm	Heavy, w/ Vitamins C & E	

4. Ayurveda - Traditional Indian Medical System, which literally means knowledge or science *(veda)* of life *(ayur),* is the traditional and ancient Indian medical system. During the colonial period of India's history when foreign interests ruled, Ayurveda was outlawed and India westernized. Recent years have seen India regain it's cultural identity and world- wide interest develop in Ayurveda. Classical Ayurvedic texts state that treating a patient effectively involves treatment of that patient as a whole - i.e. treating their consciousness, mind, and body. Ayurveda seeks to establish internal balance or "homeostasis" within the patient. The foundation of the balance is three organizing principals known as "doshas". Disease is related to an imbalance in the doshas. In functional terms, the three doshas (Vata, Pitta, and Kapha) are (respectively) associated with *motion, energy production,* and *structure.* "Vata" is the dosha that is expressed in all motion, functionally associated with activities of the locomotor system, circulation of the blood, contractions of the heart and lungs, peristalsis, elimination, and cellular transport functions. Vata is of great importance in all homeostatic mechanisms. In the natural world, Vata is expressed in *wind* and in the *movement* of water. In the human body, the seats of Vata are the large intestine, pelvic cavity, bones, skin, ears, and thighs. Vata is considered the "lead" dosha because of its quality of mobility or motion. "Pitta" is the dosha that is expressed in metabolic activities and processes involving energy exchange. Pitta is associated with glandular activities - hormone production and digestion. In the natural world, Pitta is expressed in sunshine and *fire.* In the human body, the seats of Pitta are the small intestine, stomach, sweat glands, blood, skin, and eyes. "Kapha" is the dosha that governs the structure and cohesion of the organism. Kapha is responsible for physical strength, tissue resilience, and proper body structure, including cellular and biochemical organization. In the natural world, Kapha is expressed in solid structural elements such as *earth* and rocks. In the human body, the seats of Kapha are the chest, lungs, and the spinal fluid, which surrounds the spinal cord. The structures of bone, muscle, and fat are also associated with Kapha.

The *Vata* body type is typically characterized by a *slender* build with prominent features, joints and veins, and cool, dry skin. Vata types are often moody, enthusiastic, imaginative and impulsive, quick to grasp new ideas and undertake new projects - but poor at completing them. Vata types may eat and sleep erratically, as their energy fluctuates. The Vata type is prone to insomnia, nervous disorders (hyperactivity and anxiety), constipation, cramps, and PMS.

The *Pitta* body type is typically of *medium* build, strength, and endurance. Pitta types are often well proportioned and easily maintain body weight. The Pitta person is usually fair, with red or blond hair, freckles, and a ruddy complexion. Pitta types have a sharp intellect, can be quite critical, and often have an explosive temper. Pitta types are efficient in their daily habits, eating and sleeping on a regular schedule. The Pitta type is prone to stomach ailments, ulcers/heartburn, hemorrhoids, acne, and perspire heavily.

The *Kapha* type is typically characterized by a solid, *heavy* and strong body with a tendency to be overweight. Kaphas have slow digestion, cool, damp, pale skin and thick oily hair. The Kapha type is generally slow to eat, slow to act, and slow to anger. They sleep long and deeply, tending to procrastinate. They can be quite stubborn. The Kapha type is prone to problems of high cholesterol, obesity, sinus ailments and allergies.

Most people are a mixture of Dosha characteristics or body types such as Vata-Pitta or Pitta-Kapha. Each person is unique and therefore has their own "constitution" which involves individual strengths and weaknesses. The Ayurvedic assessment or diagnosis is used to determine the patient's type or constitution. *Ayurvedic Diagnostic techniques* include detailed history taking, observation and palpation with particular attention to the (12) pulses, tongue, eyes, nails, hair, skin and urine.

Once a diagnosis has been made, the *Ayurvedic Treatment* plan will typically include four treatment methods that are designed to bring balance or homeostasis to the patient. These four main treatment methods or forms are *Cleansing & Detoxification* (Shodan), *Palliation* (Shaman), *Rejuvenation* (Rasayana) and *Mental Hygiene / Spiritual Healing* (Satvajaya). The major modalities used to facilitate these methods include the use of Diet, Herbs, Massage (primarily, with medicated oils & ghee), Sunlight, Exercise, Breathing, and Meditation.

5. Bindegewebsmassage - Connective Tissue Massage developed by Elisabeth Dicke; she discovered that certain areas on the body surface relate to certain viscera and that any imbalance affects the entire system, especially the autonomic & central nervous system, as well as hormonal systems. The strokes follow the direction of the dermatomes and affect the connective tissue. Exact strokes and systematic application are used for various pathological conditions.

6. Cranio-sacral - Developed by William Sutherland and researched by John Upledger, both osteopathic physicians. Their techniques are usually integrated with other bodywork. This work is a *somatic* approach because of the effect it has on the autonomic nervous system. It discharges high sympathetic tone, raises parasympathetic tone (relaxation), and has a positive effect on soft tissue disorders. It utilizes the breath and intuition. This work concentrates on the dura, arachnoid, and pia meningeal membranes, which surround the central nervous system. The practitioner is trained to evaluate the *motility* (rhythmic response) of this system. Cranio-sacral work involves gently guiding and releasing tensions through very mild pressure, and is claimed to be effective in treating headaches, facial pain, lower back pain, and relieving stress by balancing the autonomic nervous system. Little research exists to support these claims.

7. Esalen Massage - Named for the Esalen Institute located in Big Sur, California, this technique is a combination of Asian and Swedish Massage, and was developed in the 1960's. Typically uses little or no draping, involves long flowing strokes, and tends to be nurturing, meditative, and trance-like.

8. Feldenkrais - Developed by Moshe Feldenkrais (1904-1984). His method consists of two branches, *Awareness Through Movement* and *Functional Integration*. Awareness had to be experienced; and therefore, participants accomplished movements and postures they thought unattainable, producing greater vitality. The bodywork attempts to offset gravity, returning a participant to an early childhood state, undoing emotional/cultural programming.

9. Hellerwork - Developed by James Heller of the U.S. Consists of deep-tissue work affecting the nervous and muscular systems, with movement re-education training and *dialogue* used to discover how life issues affect emotions. Treatments are offered in ll week sessions.

10. Integrated/Eclectic Massage - Uses various bodywork techniques.

11. Jin Shin Do - A form of acupressure/shiatsu developed by Iona Teeguarden in the 1970's. The application of the pressure is longer than in Shiatsu, lasting from one to five minutes and applied to *acupoints* to reduce physical and emotional stress. This method incorporates acupressure techniques, breathing exercises, Taoist philosophy, and modern psychology.

12. Kinesiology - The study of body movement. Attention is focused on the individual muscles or groups of muscles and the specific movements they perform. *"Applied Kinesiology," Precision Muscle Testing & Touch for Health* are subjective diagnostic systems, which were derived from the work of George Goodhart D.C. Each involves isolated muscle testing and the assumption that a dysfunction of muscle, organ, tissue, or mental/emotional process will be revealed through a weakness in a specific muscle. The system is therefore purportedly used to diagnose energetic imbalances in the body and determine exactly what remedy would be most appropriate at that time. *"Three In One"* and *"Body Talk"* are recent spin-offs of *"Applied Kinesiology."* No research exists to support claims.

13. Lomi-Lomi - First reported by early travelers to the South Pacific, this massage system uses very large, broad movements. It is similar to Swedish, but uses prayer and the acknowledgment of a higher power as part of the technique.

14. Manual Lymph Drainage - Dr. Emil Vodder, Ph.D., developed this technique, which uses light compression and stroking. The manual pumping (compression) technique causes tiny lymphatic capillaries to open and close, facilitating the flow of lymph. A myotatic response propels the lymph through larger lymphatic vessels. Light strokes promote the movement of superficial lymph, and deeper strokes move lymph through the deeper vessels. MLD also stimulates the venous capillaries to absorb more material, especially excess fluid from tissue space. MLD may be useful in healthy people who have sustained injury, surgery, or who have chronic inflammation; it may be useful for people with damaged lymph vessels due to surgery, radiation therapy, injury, or congenital defects. A typical MLD session begins with light compression to the right side of the neck (superior to the clavicle) followed by gliding strokes. This sequence is repeated to the right chest area, axillary region, and right arm. The MLD session then moves to the left side of the neck, left chest area, axillary region, and arm. The MLD session then moves to the abdomen, anterior legs, posterior legs, and concludes with the back. Compression and Gliding strokes (centripetal in direction) begin with the most proximal part of limb and progress to more distal areas. Studies suggest that MLD is an effective modality for the treatment of Lymphedema (when compared to vaso-pneumatic devices) only when used in conjunction with therapeutic wrapping and when performed several times each week.

15. Movement therapy - Techniques that use awareness and movement re-education, in combination with other massage manipulations. (See: Alexander, Feldenkrais, Ortho-Bionomy and Tai Chi)

16. Muscle Energy Technique *(MET)* was developed in the early 20th century by T.J. Ruddy and Fred Mitchell (both Osteopathic physicians). Muscle Energy Technique involves the voluntary contraction of muscle in a precisely controlled direction, at varying levels of intensity, against a distinctly executed counterforce applied by the operator. MET is classified as an active technique, in which the patient contributes the corrective force. MET is used to lengthen a shortened, contracted, or spastic muscle or to strengthen a weakened muscle. Proponents' state that MET may also provide relief for passive congestion, localized edema, and restricted range of motion.

17. Myofascial Release - *(*MFR) is a term first used by Robert Ward, D.O., in the 1960's and later (1980's) adopted by John Barnes, a physical therapist, to describe his method of treating the facial system. MFR builds upon the inherent tissue motion and fluid-like nature of fibrous connective tissue. Fascia including the collagenous component and ground substance (matrix) should be markedly fluid-like *(sol or solvent)* to allow for proper movement. Trauma, stress, and inflammation may cause this fascia to solidify (become *gel-like*), shorten, and possibly adhere to other tissue, causing painful restrictions. Fascia surrounds every system of the body. MFR technique applies prolonged light pressure without movement, but with specific direction. The tissue warms, causing the matrix of the fascia to return to its more fluid *(solvent)* state, releasing the restrictions. Skin rolling is also used to loosen superficial fascia and prepare the tissue for deeper myofascial work.

18. Neuromuscular Technique *(NMT)* was developed by Stanley Leif, a natural healer born in Latvia in the 1890's. Janet Travell, M.D., is credited with giving scientific credence to the therapy. Bonnie Prudden brought NMT to the practice of massage with her book *Pain Erasure.* In NMT, the body's loss of mobility and accompanying pain, caused by trauma, disease, stress, postural deviations, or poor nutrition, are seen as affecting other areas of the body, which compensate for these restrictions, causing *more* neuromuscular dysfunction. NMT identifies the areas of abnormality, manipulates the tissue and tendonous attachments to normalize function. NMT utilizes Travell's trigger point work to identify areas where pain is being referred. NMT uses: *gliding, ischemic compression, skin rolling, and stretching* to interrupt the pathophysiological reflex arc at the sight of the injury and referral areas (via Gate Theory mechanisms) subsides, allowing the muscle to relax and return the reflex arc to normal activity. Manipulation of the associated muscle spindle cells and Golgi tendon organs are also accomplished with these techniques to further normalization of neuro-muscular activity.

19. Polarity Therapy - Developed by Dr. Randolph Stone in the mid 1900's, this technique derived from both Eastern and Western practices, emphasizes energy-flow, emotional tension and/or pain release. It uses exercise, nutrition, and *love* (*the foremost principle*), as well as gentle bodywork to balance the positive and negative energies, and free the flow of energy throughout the body. The Polarity therapist works to balance energy within the channels/meridians and energy centers (Chakras) of the recipient. Five-element theory (see shiatsu) also plays a role in polarity. Beginning polarity students are taught 22 basic movements to balance the entire body. These basic movements include such techniques as: the *Cradle, Neck Stretch, Tummy Rock, Leg Pull, Ankle Press, Pelvis & Knee Rock, Arm Rotation, Elbow Milk, Occipital Press, and Brushing Off.*

20. Positional Release - Originally developed by Lawrence Jones, D. O., and known as Strain-Counterstrain technique, this method involves moving the joint and affected muscle into a position of maximum comfort, holding it there for an appropriate period of time, and then *very slowly* returning it to its normal resting position. Pain is relieved by shortening the contracted muscle and putting mild strain on its antagonist, which through reflex action will result in the shortened muscle being relaxed by reducing inappropriate proprioceptor activity.

21. Postural Integration - Developed by Jack Painter, this technique uses manipulation, bioenergetics, acupressure, breath-work, and dialogue. Both P.I. and Structural Integration are related to Rolfing.

22. Proprioceptive Neuromuscular Facilitation (*PNF*) - Uses stretching to improve the mobility of joints. These stretches often require the assistance of a partner. Contract-relax techniques are used. The muscle is comfortably lengthened until resistance is met. Then the client performs an isometric contraction of that muscle against resistance for 5-10 seconds. The LMT passively moves the body part through the gained range until comfortable resistance is again met and this action is repeated until the desired gain is obtained. The neurological phenomena of "*Post-Isometric Relaxation*" and "*Reciprocal Inhibition*" explain the results gained from PNF.

23. Reflexology - Developed by William Fitzgerald and originally called *Zone Therapy*, (also from the work of Eunice Ingham), this technique is based upon the theory that pressure applied to specific areas of the feet (may include areas on the hands and head) stimulates corresponding areas in distant areas of the body. Most reflexologists focus on the reflex points of the feet and hands. Firm pressure (*Thumb walking, Finger Walking, Hook and Backup*) with the thumb (or finger) is applied to specific nerve endings in the appendages, creating a reflex response in body organs and tissues, and normalizing function. Research supports its efficacy.

24. Reiki - Founded by Dr. Mikao Usui, this technique is based on the principles of Chi or universal life energy. Reiki promotes healing through methods that are rooted in *spiritual* tradition. The practitioner places his/her hands very gently on a person's head, chest, abdomen, and back. Practitioners go through three levels of training or attunements. Reiki, as noted above, is the gentle "energetic" hands-on technique of accessing and directing Ki (Qi, Chi, Prana, Life-Force Energy, etc.) into the lives of others. The word Reiki (pronounced ray-key) means "universal life energy." Reiki students experience attunement by taking Reiki classes that allow them to "channel higher amounts of Ki." Reiki students are empowered by Reiki "masters" to experience attunement.

Reiki techniques involve the laying on of hands, visualization, symbols, and meditative practices to direct energy (Ki, the universal life force) from the *Hara* (center of gravity) which is located below the navel (consciously) through the body's various energy centers or *Chakras*. Self-treatment is also possible using Reiki techniques, creating balance, and facilitating healing on all levels; Physical, Mental, Emotional, and Spiritual. Benefits claimed from Reiki therapy include an increased awareness, creativity, vitality and energy, the promotion of healing, pain reduction, the promotion of a loving and gentle spirit, stress reduction, and the removal of energy and emotional blocks.

Chakras & Relationships

Name	Number	Color	Sound	Purpose/Function	Element
Crown	7	Violet or White		Divine Understanding	Thought
Third Eye	6	Indigo	Aum (om)	Inner Vision	Light
Throat	5	Blue	Hung	Wisdom, Judgment	Sound
Heart	4	Green	Yung	Love	Air
Solar Plexus	3	Yellow	Rung	Emotions	Fire
Sexual	2	Orange	Vung	Relationships	Water
Root/ Base	1	Red	Lung	Physical Body	Earth

Symbols are given as a part of the Reiki II attunement and are used to increase power, for emotional healing, and for absentee or distance healing.

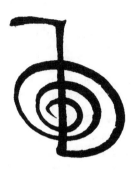 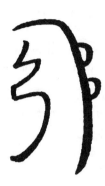 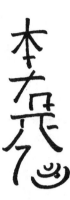

1st REIKI SYMBOL   **2nd REIKI SYMBOL**   **3rd REIKI SYMBOL**

25. Rolfing - Developed by Ida Rolf, a biochemist, this method of structural integration attempts to bring the physical structures of the body into alignment around a central axis, producing physical and psychological balance. It is a *deep* connective tissue massage, attempting to reshape the body's physical posture and to realign the muscular and connective tissue. Rolfing attempts to lift and lengthen the body's trunk creating a sense of lightness and greater mobility. It is usually performed in a series of at least 10 treatments. Rolfing was first known as Structural Integration.

26. Shiatsu - Means finger pressure. Shiatsu is also called Acupressure and is a traditional Asian healing method systematized in the early 1900's in Japan, but which has Chinese origins dating TO 2500 B.C. This modality views a healthy body as one in which the energy (**Chi, Ki, or Qi**) is balanced and free flowing through 14 invisible channels called **meridians**. Chi manifests itself as five interrelated elements of energy - *fire, earth, metal, water, and wood*. All are created from these elements, and humans are influenced by a combination of all five. When the vital energy becomes *imbalanced* or stagnated, the body develops disorders. *Balance* has to be restored to allow the body to correct the problem. The energy stagnates along the channels at points called *tsubo*. **Pain and tenderness** of a (ashi) point indicates stagnation or **imbalance** of Chi (or blood). Traditional Chinese Medicine (TCM) considers illness to be an *imbalance* between Yin and Yang, the Five Elements, or external influences. In diagnosing an illness, one considers the above characteristics, as well as qualities of the pulse, the condition of the tongue, and by palpating the abdomen *(hara)*. Finger, palm, or foot pressure is sequentially applied to the channels and points (tsubos) to manipulate energy and bring about a balance of energy, and in turn, health.

The following charts list some commonly used points, their locations, and indications:

Point	Location	Indications
LU-7	On the radial aspect of the forearm, proximal to styloid process of the radius.	Headache, neck pain, cough, asthma, facial paralysis,
LU-9	On the wrist crease, in the depression between the radial artery and the abductor pollicis longus tendon.	Cough, asthma, shortness of breath, pain in wrist & shoulder
LI-4	On dorsum of hand, between 1st & 2nd metacarpal bones, at midpoint of 2nd bone and close to its radial border.	Common cold, headache, toothache, swelling of face, nosebleed, TMJ, all pain in body, colds, sore throat, asthma, labor problems, insomnia
LI-11	At the elbow, midway between the bicep brachii tendon and the lateral epicondyle of the humerus.	Fever, skin diseases, hypertension, sore throat, fever, colds, toothache, shoulder and arm pain, & paralysis,
LI-15	In the depression anterior and inferior to acromion, at the origin of the deltoid muscle.	Disorders of shoulder, elbow and the surrounding tissues, hemiplegia
LI-20	In the naso-labial groove, at the level of midpoint of lateral border of ala nasi.	Nasal congestion (rhinitis), loss of sense of smell, sinusitis, Bell's Palsy, parasites
ST-7	At the lower border of the zygomatic arch, in the depression anterior to the condyloid process of the mandible.	Benefits ears, jaw, teeth, toothache, TMJ, Trigeminal Neuralgia, Bell's Palsy, gum disorders,
ST-36	Below the knee, 3-cun inferior to lower border of patella and one finger-breadth lateral to anterior crest of tibia.	All stomach disorders, nausea/vomiting, shock, seizure, headache, neurosis, allergies, fever, hip & leg pain, edema, hemiplegia
SP-6	Medial side of lower leg, 3-cun superior to prominence of medial malleolus, in depression close to crest of tibia.	Insomnia, digestive, gynecological & urinary disorders (enuresis & retention), impotence, edema, neurasthenia,
SP-9	Medial side of leg, in the depression formed by the medial condyle of the tibia & the posterior border of the tibia.	Promotes urination, knee disorders, edema, and abdominal distention
HT-7	At the wrist, on radial side of flexor carpi ulnaris, in depression at proximal border of pisiform bone.	"Shen Men" (calm the spirit), insomnia, heart palpitations, and poor memory
SI-3	On ulnar border of hand in the substantial depression, proximal to the head of the 5th metacarpal bone.	Stiffness & pain in neck and upper back, seizures, occipital headache, tinnitus, deafness, low back pain, depression, malaria
BL-23	1.5 cun later to the lower border of the L-2 vertebrae.	Edema, irregular menses, seminal emission, and urinary system disorders
BL-40	At the back of the knee, on the popliteal crease, in the depression midway between the tendons of biceps femoris and semitendinosus.	Lumbar pain, sciatica, hip and knee pain, leg cramps, skin diseases, heat stroke, seizures, gastrointestinal & urinary system disorders
BL-60	Behind the ankle joint, in the depression between the prominence of the lateral malleolus and the Achilles tendon.	Lumbar pain, sciatica, knee, ankle and heel pain, cramps & paralysis, cough, difficult labor
BL-62	On the foot, 0.5-cun inferior to inferior border of lateral malleolus, in depression posterior to the peroneal tendons.	Chills & fever, dizziness, Headache, eye disorders, stiffness in the neck and back
KI-1	Between the 2nd & 3rd metatarsal bones, one third of the distance between the base of the 2nd toe and the heel.	Lowest point of body, headache, fear, hypertension, and dizziness

KI-3	In the depression between the medial malleolus and the Achilles tendon, level with prominence of the malleolus.	Throat, intestines, teeth, ears, cough, asthma, lumbar pain, cold limbs
PC-6	On the forearm, 2-cun proximal to wrist crease, between the tendons of the palmaris longus and flexor carpi radialis.	Motion sickness, palpitations, nausea, vomiting, insomnia, hiccups, chest congestion, abdominal pain
SJ-5	On the lateral forearm, 2-cun proximal to wrist crease, in the depression between the radius and ulna, on the radial side of the extensor digitorum communis tendons.	Common cold, headache, eye and ear disorders, constipation, stiffness of the neck, shoulder and back
SJ-17	Behind the earlobe, between the ramus of the mandible and the mastoid process.	Deafness, tinnitus, ear disorders, Bell's Palsy, pain of teeth and gums
GB-20	Midway between the external occipital protuberance and mastoid process, in the hollow between the origins of the sternocleidomastoid and trapezius muscles.	Tension & migraine headache, stiff neck, hypertension, common cold, eye and ear disorders (tinnitus), dizziness, vertigo, Bell's Palsy
GB-21	Midway between the 7th cervical vertebrae and the tip of the acromion, at the crest of the trapezius muscle.	Stiff neck and upper back with pain & neuropathy, cough, breast pain, prolonged labor, poor lactation, uterine bleeding and mastitis, and hyperthyroidism
GB-30	One third of the distance between the prominence of the greater trochanter and the sacro-coccygeal hiatus.	Sciatica, disorders of hip and low back including pain, lower extremity paralysis,
GB-34	Below the lateral aspect of the knee, in the tender depression 1 cun anterior, and inferior to head of the fibula.	Tendon disorders, sciatica, liver/gall bladder diseases, bitter taste in mouth with reflux, vertigo, lateral lower extremity pain, hemiplegia
LV-3	On the dorsum of the foot, in the depression distal to the junction of the 1st & 2nd metatarsal bones.	Headache, vertigo, seizure, insomnia, blurred vision, menstrual, urinary & genital disorders
DU-14	On the midline at the base of the neck, in the depression below the spinous process of the 7th cervical vertebrae.	Common cold, chills, fever, stiffness in spine, night sweats
DU-20	Along midline of head, in depression 5-cun posterior to anterior hairline and 7 cun superior to posterior hairline.	Nourish the brain, hypertension, calms the spirit, headache, prolapse of rectum or uterus
DU-26	Above the upper lip, one third of the distance down from the nose on the midline.	Heat stroke, shock, seizure, Bell's Palsy, lumbar pain, benefits nose and face,
REN-12	On the midline of the abdomen, 4-cun above the umbilicus.	All disease of the stomach and spleen, anxiety, over-thinking
Yin Tang	At the glabella, at the midpoint between the medial extremities of the eyebrows.	Headache, disorders of the nose and eyes, dizziness/vertigo, insomnia, calms the spirit
Tai Yang	At the temple, in the tender depression 1-cun posterior to the midpoint between the lateral extremity of the eyebrow and the outer canthus of the eye.	Migraines, dizziness, Trigeminal Neuralgia, toothache, Bell's Palsy, disorders of the eye and mouth

27. Soma - Working with the fascia and musculature, the Soma practitioner attempts to restore circulation and original perfection to the body. The holographic body reading recognizes that each individual has a unique blueprint. Soma is related to Somatic Therapy, Hokomi Bodywork, and Lomi Lomi.

28. Sports Massage - Athletic training programs include massage to enhance performance and prevent or rehabilitate injuries. The techniques used depend on the timing of the massage and the intent.

> **a.** *Pre-event:* Stimulate circulation, warm tissue, calm nervous tension and prepare athlete for maximum performance (light gliding, compression, palmar friction, & lifting and broadening). Avoid areas of tenderness.

> **b.** *Post-event:* Relieve soreness, sedate, and assist in re-establishing circulation and removing metabolic by-products. (Gliding; compression; circular friction; easy stretching; lifting and broadening along with passive ROM and easy stretching.) *Precautions* for Post Event:

>> **1)** *Hyperthermia* - *Heat* production exceeds heat loss - Symptoms: Clumsiness, excessive sweating, headache, nausea, and dizziness. The *degree* of severity depends on what symptoms are present. Heat cramps can be caused by dehydration. Encourage hydration and use reciprocal inhibition techniques to *relieve cramping*. Heat exhaustion is more *severe*. The athlete's skin will be cool and pale, profuse sweating, chills, nausea. In this case *refer* to a medical unit. *Heat stroke* is the most severe. The athlete may be incoherent, exhibit acute confusion or aggression and their skin will be dry. *Refer* to medical unit *immediately*.

>> **2)** *Hypothermia* - Heat loss exceeds heat production - Symptoms: shivering, euphoria and may appear intoxicated. Encourage hot drinks and keep warm. Talk to the athlete and observe; if it is an extreme case, refer to medical unit.

>> **3)** *Strains and Sprains* - Strain refers to damaged muscles or tendons, and sprain refers to damaged ligaments. Sprains are classified or graded as:
>> *Grade One* - *mild,* 0-20% fiber tear, holds against resistance; may be tender & swollen, normal post event techniques O.K.
>> *Grade Two* - *moderate,* 20-75% tear, will show increased laxity with moderate resistance, some edema, muscle splinting.
>> *Grade Three* - *severe,* 75-100% tear, unstable, painful to touch, function altered, requires immediate medical attention; **refer** to medical unit for RICE & treatment. Second and third level sprains/strains can be identified by increased pain and instability in the injured area when stress/stretching/resistance applied.

Make sure the athlete has cooled down, and replenished fluids prior to the massage. Get feedback and watch for signs of exhaustion and spasm. Be aware of any blisters and contusions, and obtain first aid if appropriate.

29. Stone Therapy - Massage with (heated or cooled) smooth, specially selected stones. Developed during the 1990's, Stone Therapy has recently gained popularity with both spas and independent practitioners. Most commonly, treatments involve the application of heated (120° F) stones to Acupressure/ Trigger Point locations or the use of the stones (with lubricant) in applying effleurage, friction, or compression techniques. Proponents claim that deep relaxation, stress reduction, detoxification, energetic balancing, and personal transformation all result from the technique. Basalt (a type of river rock) appears to be the stone of choice, in that it has a smooth surface and desirable thermal characteristics. Precious and semi- precious stones are also used upon corresponding Charka sites. The stones should be properly sanitized after each use.

30. Structural Integration - See Rolfing and Postural Integration. Structural Integration was the name first given to the process now known as Rolfing.

31. Therapeutic Touch - The "laying on of hands" technique was developed by Dolores Krieger, Ph.D., R.N. *Gentle and non-invasive*, it works on and **above** the body (touching is not necessary), using a meditative process and dispersing blocked energy, allowing the practitioner to channel healing energy to the client. Recent research suggests its efficacy in specific cases.

32. Trager - Developed by Milton Trager M.D. This approach is not so much a technique but a way of **relearning**--allowing the body to re-educate itself through movement. The Trager Method uses gentle rocking and shaking. The movement of muscles, limbs, and joints to produce experiences of lightness, freedom, and ease. Reducing tension is the goal. Trager uses "*hook up*"- a state of awareness on the part of the practitioner. *Mentastics*, a word for mental gymnastics, is also taught in each session. These experiences affect the central nervous system and proprioceptors, causing relaxation of the muscles and increased mobility.

33. Trigger Point Therapy - A trigger point is an area of hyperirritability. The pain that arises in a trigger point is also felt at a distance (*referral pattern*). Sensory and motor phenomena, such as pain, tenderness, spasm, numbness, and tingling are felt at the referral area. **Dr. Janet Travell** has done extensive research and writing in this field, her two-volume text: *Myofascial Pain & Dysfunction* (1992) is considered to be the ultimate reference. These points are painful to the touch and are associated with dysfunctional neurological *reflex arcs*. Deactivating these trigger points by active stretching and direct pressure (injection and Spray & Stretch technique) reduces the pain and improves the function of the areas involved. Bonnie Pruden is the massage therapist most associated with Trigger Point Therapy. She is the author of *Pain Erasure* (1980) and *Myotherapy* (1984), which describe in detail techniques similar to those of NMT.

34. Tui Na – Chinese Medical Massage, literally translated means "push" and "hold." Tui Na (also tuina) arises from the most ancient Asian massage technique "Anmo" (press and rub) which was in use for year's prior, but was first named about 200 B.C. The term "Tui Na" was first used in the Tang Dynasty in about 1300 A.D. During the 6th century (A.D.) Traditional Chinese Medicine (TCM) spread to Japan and Korea where Anma and Amma were (respectively) developed. Shiatsu grew from traditional Anma therapy in Japan about 1915. There is some evidence that Portuguese missionaries brought Tui Na teaching manuals home from China in the 17th century, providing the basis for European development of Swedish Remedial Gymnastics and later Swedish massage.

Tui Na incorporates the concepts of Yin and Yang, Five Element Theory, 14 Channels & points and of Chi. Diagnosis is by: Looking, Asking, Listening/Smelling, and Touching. Tongue and Pulse diagnosis are also incorporated. Techniques are used to harmonize channels, balance Chi, normalize Yin & Yang, and to tonify or sedate. Techniques used include: Pushing, Grasping, Pressing, Rubbing, Kneading, Tapping (dotting), Rolling, Pinching, Nipping, Pulling, Knocking, Scratching, Chopping, Pounding, and a multitude of variations.

The thumb, fingers, hand, forearm, elbow, and numerous devices are used by the practitioner in the application of techniques. Gua Sha (scraping with a spoon or another flat instrument), Cupping (applying suction with a glass cup or jar), and the application of Moxa (infrared heat from burning herbs) are also examples of traditional Tui Na techniques. Various massage "clubs" or tools are often used to substitute for the hands & fingers of the therapist. Both soft and osseous tissues are manipulated in traditional Tui Na, with the traditional Tui Na therapist (doctor) receiving many years of specialized training.

35. Watsu - Water based technique developed by Harold Dull at Harbin Hot Springs, CA. in the 1980's. Watsu incorporates the thermal effects and buoyancy of water emersion with bodywork elements of Shiatsu, European massage and movement therapy to bring receivers into "sync." Neutral temperature water (96° F), breath work, support *(cradling),* and gentle movement allow the receiver to reach a heightened state of awareness and relaxation. The receiver is "floated" through a series of positions, stretches are facilitated and (acupressure) points are stimulated. Proponents claim improvements in posture, increased range of motion, improved muscle tone, decreased (chronic) pain, and speeding of the healing (both physical and emotional) process. Dull is the author of *Watsu: Freeing the Body in Water*. Training and certification are offered through the Worldwide Aquatic Bodywork Association.

Review Questions - Massage/Bodywork Theory, Assessment, & Practice

1. Chi manifests itself as five interrelated elements of cosmological energy. Circle the *incorrect* element of Traditional Chinese Medicine:
    a) Fire
    b) Earth
    c) Wind
    d) Water

2. Your client has a subacute ankle sprain. What is the ***best*** stroke to facilitate recovery of this type of injury?
    a) Gliding
    b) Deep compression
    c) Transverse friction
    d) Vibration

3. Your client has psoriasis on his back. He desires a full body massage. What is the most appropriate course of action?
    a) Explain that psoriasis is contagious and you must reschedule the massage
    b) Ask them to cleanse the area thoroughly with bacterial soap and massage the area
    c) Complete the massage, but avoid the affected area
    d) None of the above

4. Your client explains that they have been diagnosed with phlebitis. What is the ***best*** response?
    a) Proceed with caution, but complete the massage, working lightly over affected area until you have time to talk to her Dr
    b) Explain that you want to research & consult with her doctor because certain conditions are contraindicated; reschedule the massage
    c) Proceed with massage, but do energy work instead of Swedish
    d) None of the above

5. Shiatsu is an ancient Oriental healing method, which includes:
    a) Balancing the Chi (energy) through invisible channels (meridians)
    b) Yin and Yang, governing forces (energy) within universe
    c) Diagnosis of illness through qualities of the pulse and condition of tongue
    d) All of the above

6. Which of the following conditions are contraindicated for massage?
    a) Abnormal lumps
    b) Acute fever
    c) Acute inflammation (i.e. phlebitis, diverticulitis, cellulitis)
    d) All of the above

7.   You suspect that your client has impetigo. What should you do?
   a) Clean the affected area with alcohol & massage the area
   b) Avoid the area and proceed with the massage
   c) Explain to the client what they need to do to treat the area
   d) Explain what you suspect and politely reschedule the massage. Suggest the client see her doctor for treatment.

8.   Your client has chronic low back problems. While prone, she complains of pain in the low back area. What should you do *first*?
   a) Place pillow under her abdomen
   b) Place more pillows under her feet
   c) Ask her to breath into the pain & it will go away
   d) None of the above

9.   Your client comes in with extremely painful whiplash. He was in an auto accident yesterday, his neck is very stiff and sore, and he thinks massage will help. What is the best course of action?
   a) Explain you cannot do deep work, but Swedish could help relax musculature and proceed with the massage
   b) Treat with NMT routine for cervical area
   c) Work the area with cross fiber friction
   d) Refer to & reschedule the massage after his consulting with the physician

10.   Circle the *incorrect* statement:
   a) Ying & Yang are opposite but complimentary forces
   b) Yin is located on the posterior body & Yang on the anterior
   c) GB2l is located midway between shoulder & C7
   d) LI20 is a point you would work for sinus & allergy conditions

11.   Kinesiology is the study of:
   a) Exercise and gentle bodywork to balance the positive & negative energies
   b) Body movement and the relationship of groups of muscles and their movement
   c) The deep fascial layers of the body
   d) Acupoints used to reduce physical & emotional stress

12.   Which of the following statements is an *incorrect* statement?
   a) Trager is a method of re-education through movement & the experiences affect the central nervous system, causing relaxation.
   b) Trigger point therapy is a gentle, energy technique quieting the nervous system.
   c) Reiki is a technique based on Chi & spiritual tradition; the practitioner gently places their hands on the client's body.
   d) Therapeutic Touch, sometimes called "laying on of hands" is gentle & non-invasive, using meditation & dispersing blocked energy, often being done above the client's body.

13. When massaging the anterior neck, what structure should be avoided?
    a) Carotid artery
    b) Internal jugular vein
    c) Vagus Nerve
    d) All of the above

14. The term Mentastics and hook-up are terms used in:
    a) Rolfing
    b) Hellerwork
    c) Trager
    d) Jin Shin Do

15. In Traditional Chinese Medicine, the organs are associated with certain elements. The organs associated with the Earth element are:
    a) Spleen & Stomach
    b) Gall Bladder & Liver
    c) Kidney and Urinary Bladder
    d) Lung and Large Intestine

16. When massaging Adductor Longus and Sartorius, what structures are to be avoided?
    a) Femoral Triangle
    b) Brachial Plexus
    c) Subclavian Artery
    d) All of the above

17. A new client does not want to complete your intake questionnaire. What is the *first* thing you should do?
    a) Refuse to work on them unless they complete the form
    b) Reschedule the session & ask them to fill the form out at home
    c) Continue to ask questions; if the client gives you all the necessary information, you proceed with the massage
    d) Proceed with the massage & ask them to fill out the form and mail it to you

18. Your client is lying in the supine position and complains of low back pain. What should you do *first*?
    a) Turn him on his side
    b) Ask him to breath into the pain & it will go away
    c) Place pillow(s) under his knees
    d) Stop the massage

19. Relaxation of contracted muscles following massage can *best* be explained by:
    a) Endorphin release
    b) The mechanical affects on muscle tone
    c) The removal of toxins from the muscle tissue
    d) The affect on nerve impulses involved in resetting muscle tone.

20. Your client has a large, dark mole on his back. You have noticed a sudden change in appearance & size. What should you do?
    a) Tell the client you think the mole may be cancerous & should have a doctor look at it immediately
    b) Do not massage the immediate area
    c) Explain to him that you have noticed a sudden change in the mole's appearance; suggest he may want to have a doctor examine it just to be on the safe side (avoid immediate area)
    d) Massage the area since moles are not contagious

21. You client has varicose veins. Circle the *incorrect* statement.
    a) Varicose veins occur when the vein is enlarged and stretched due to prolonged back pressure in the vein
    b) Massage proximal to the area is not contraindicated, but obtain Dr.'s OK
    c) It is O.K. to massage the area if you use very light, gliding strokes
    d) Varicose veins occur mainly in the superficial leg veins

22. Range of Motion is **best** determined by:
    a) Joint movement assessments
    b) Palpation of the affected area
    c) Myofascial release techniques
    d) Stretching

23. The mechanical effects of massage include:
    a) Disruption of adhesions & stretching the muscle
    b) Increased cellular metabolism
    c) Reduction in pain by affecting the nervous system
    d) Reduction in noxious stimulation of the nervous system, lowering stress

24. A therapist must be concerned with personal hygiene at all times. The **most** important hygiene habit is:
    a) Unscented deodorant
    b) Oral hygiene
    c) Clean hands and nails
    d) Professional image

25. The **primary** goal of post-event sports massage is to:
    a) Re-establish circulation which aids in recovery from negative affects of activity
    b) Stimulate circulation
    c) Warm tissue
    d) Calm nervous tension

26. Massage would be indicated for:
    a) Post-acute bursitis
    b) Acute whiplash
    c) Arteriosclerosis
    d) Lyme Disease

27. Massage affects the body in a number of ways. Circle the *incorrect* statement.
    a) Massage increases cell metabolism and hastens healing.
    b) Massage interrupts noxious stimulation to nerve activity and helps reduce pain.
    c) Massage breaks up and reduces cellulite.
    d) Massage affects neurological and chemical activity causing arteriolar and capillary dilation, increased skin temperature, and localized skin hyperemia.

28. The *most* widely recognized physiological effect of massage is:
    a) Reduction in stress
    b) Relaxation
    c) Improvement in the condition of the skin
    d) Increase in blood and lymph circulation

29. Your client complains of a muscle cramp in her Gastrocnemius. Select the treatment which is *useful* in reducing muscle cramping?
    a) Light vibration to the muscle and surrounding area to quiet the nerves
    b) Tapotement
    c) Unassisted stretching of affected muscle
    d) Reciprocal Inhibition stretching technique

30. Massage can reduce stress; the reduction in stress can be contributed to:
    Circle the incorrect statement.
    a) The affect it has on the nervous system and over stimulated nerve activity.
    b) The individual's psychological state & its effect on nociceptive impulses.
    c) The reduction of sympathetic activity.
    d) The reduction of parasympathetic activity.

31. Delayed muscle soreness can result from sporadic exercise activities. Circle the incorrect statement.
    a) It may be the result of trauma to microscopic muscle filaments.
    b) Massage can reduce recovery time through improved circulation & removal of metabolic by-products.
    c) Massage can prevent fibrosis.
    d) Massage removes the build up of lactic acid in the tissue.

32. All soft tissue is controlled by the:
    a) Circulatory system
    b) Muscular system
    c) Nervous system
    d) Immune system

33. Before massaging, the physician's recommendation is extremely important in certain conditions, which include:
    a) Circulatory problems.
    b) Cancer
    c) Herniated disc
    d) All of the above

34. Psychological effects of massage include:
    a) Increased cellular metabolism
    b) Localized skin hyperemia
    c) Increase in skin temperature
    d) None of the above

35. Tapotement should not be used over the:
    a) Gluteal area
    b) Upper lumbar, inferior to ribs
    c) Posterior lower extremities
    d) Thoracic area

36. When massaging an injured limb, you should start:
    a) Proximal to the injury
    b) Distal to the injury
    c) Over the injury
    d) None of the above

37. When massaging your client's upper extremities, what area(s) should be avoided?
    a) Cubital area of elbow
    b) Medial brachium
    c) Ulnar notch of elbow
    d) All of the above

38. Tapotement (percussive) techniques are described below: Circle the incorrect description.
    a) Hacking/cupping
    b) Slapping/tapping
    c) Pincement/beating
    d) Chucking/popping

39. Massage can reduce pain by:
    a) Affecting the cause - nociceptive stimulation
    b) Affecting the processing of noxious stimulation
    c) Affecting the conduction of pain impulses
    d) All of the above

40. Ice massage is effective in reducing pain because:
    a) It affects the conduction of pain impulses.
    b) It alters the processing of pain impulses.
    c) It acts directly on the source of the pain reducing noxious stimulation.
    d) All of the above.

41. Your client suffers from emphysema.   Massage may:
    a) Temporarily reduce anxiety/stress due to changes in the client's breathing.
    b) Relax contracted musculature of the accessory muscles which become
       involved with assisting breathing.
    c) Temporarily increase rib-cage mobility by relaxing intercostals.
    d) All of the above.

42. Which of the following statements is incorrect?
    a) There are five basic massage strokes.
    b) Pressure strokes should follow the venous flow (centripetal).
    c) Light vibration is the best stroke for stimulating the tissue.
    d) Tapotement is the best stroke for stimulating the tissue.

43. Your client has edema and has a doctor's OK for massage. Your treatment plan
    would use which of the following strokes:
    a) Tapotement
    b) Kneading
    c) Fast, rhythmical gliding
    d) Slow, rhythmical gliding

44. The most widely used massage stroke is:
    a) Kneading
    b) Vibration
    c) Gliding
    d) Tapotement

45. Fibromyalgia may be best treated by:
    a) Connective tissue massage (myofascial release, friction, kneading)
    b) Light vibration
    c) Percussive strokes
    d) None of the above

46.	Circle the *incorrect* answer. The purpose of gliding strokes is to:
a)	Stretch the fascia
b)	Determine your client's pain tolerance
c)	Evaluate the client's soft tissue
d)	Enhance venous blood & lymphatic flow

47.	The best stroke to free adhesions in the muscle belly is:
a)	Friction
b)	Kneading
c)	Gliding
d)	Tapotement

48.	Friction is:
a)	Primarily used to reach deeper tissue, especially around the joint spaces and bony prominances
b)	Often beneficial in post-event sports massage
c)	The primary stroke used to re-establishing circulation
d)	Only applied perpendicular to the muscle fiber

49.	Passive joint movement includes:
a)	Having the client participate by contracting the muscles involved
b)	Having the client perform a motion with the assistance of the therapist
c)	Having the client remain relaxed while the therapist stretches & moves the body part
d)	None of the above

50.	When evaluating Range of Motion, you ask your client to rotate his head as far to the right as he can. This type of movement is considered to be:
a.	Passive
b.	Active resisted
c.	Active
d.	PNF

51.	Your client has tight, shortened leg muscles from cycling. Cycling is his primary form of exercise. You would recommend which of the following activities:
a)	Meditation
b)	Weight training
c)	Aerobics
d)	Yoga

52. Reciprocal inhibition is a form of stretching which requires the client to:
    a) Remain passive while the therapist completes the stretch and movement
    b) Bouncing or bobbing force used with body momentum to achieve the desired stretch
    c) Body part is moved to point where tension is experienced & held for 10 seconds; the individual contracts the muscle being stretched against resistance for 5 seconds & then the muscle is stretched further
    d) Contract the antagonist to muscle being stretched, allowing the muscle being stretched to relax

53. Your client is an amputee. The recommended stroke for treating the stump is:
    a) Vibration
    b) Tapotement
    c) Friction
    d) Gliding

54. Your client is suffering from lymphedema as a result of post-operative trauma & bed rest. Massage can reduce edema in this situation because the results can produce:
    a) Movement of the edema fluid from the tissues to the blood
    b) An increase in urine output
    c) An increase in blood flow to the area
    d) All of the above

55. Your client has high blood pressure, and her doctor recommended massage to reduce anxiety. Which stroke would you use to help lower blood pressure?
    a) Vibration
    b) Petrissage
    c) Deep gliding
    d) Slow gliding

56. The Femoral Triangle is an endangerment site. Certain anatomical structures are located in this area. Circle the incorrect statement.
    a) Sartorius, Adductor Longus, & Inguinal Ligament border this area
    b) Femoral nerve, artery, and vein located in this area
    c) Great Saphenous vein & lymph nodes located in this area
    d) Basilic Vein located in this area

57. When applying friction, the therapist should:
    a) Penetrate the tissue gradually and release gradually
    b) Keep her thumbs in alignment with the wrists
    c) Apply pressure from her body, not just the thumbs
    d) All of the above

58. A therapist's body mechanics is extremely important in preventing injury, body fatigue, and muscle strain. Circle the *incorrect* statement.
   a) A therapist should bend knees & keep back straight.
   b) Good body mechanics, while important to the therapist's well-being, really do not affect the massage itself.
   c) Hands & elbows should remain close to the body, with shoulders and wrists relaxed.
   d) Proper balance on both feet, with knees flexed & using legs, pelvis, & torso to provide the required leverage, gives the therapist the strength needed to apply pressure.

59. As a therapist, you injure your wrist. What should you do?
   a) RICE as needed. Rest until injury is healed
   b) Correct your body mechanics when massaging
   c) Use flexibility & strengthening exercises as a preventive measure
   d) All of the above

60. Client intake forms are extremely important. The *most* important reason is:
   a) Careful notes help you assess and develop a treatment plan
   b) Information received gives you medical history and helps recognize any contraindications or precautions
   c) To get to know your client and specific needs
   d) Obtaining all necessary client information can help protect the therapist if there is a malpractice suit

61. During a massage, your client's feedback includes:
   a) Changes in breathing patterns
   b) Flinching or tightening of muscles
   c) Verbal feedback
   d) All of the above

62. Myofascial release is a specialized massage technique which:
   a) Is applied by prolonged, light pressure
   b) Often uses skin rolling to prepare the tissue
   c) Warms the tissue & releases restrictions between layers of connective tissue
   d) All of the above

63. Your client tells you they have been feeling extremely fatigued for the past week and running a low-grade fever. He thinks massage can help with the fatigue.
   a) Proceed with Swedish for relaxation
   b) Question him and attempt to determine what is causing his fatigue and recommend a treatment
   c) Get more information before preceding with the massage
   d) Explain to client that you must reschedule the massage & refer to appropriate health care professional

64. Massage of paralyzed limbs is beneficial because:
a) It helps reduce the flaccidness.
b) It helps restore nerve activity to limb.
c) It improves blood circulation to the limb.
d) All of the above.

65. Facial massage and pressure applied to LI-20 may help improve:
a) Wrinkles
b) Sinus and congestion
c) Beautify condition of skin
d) All of the above

66. Deep compressive strokes result in:
a) Increased circulation & hyperemia
b) Reduction of lactic acid
c) Stimulation
d) Tone muscle

67. Endangerment sites are:
a) Areas which warrant special precautions
b) Areas with underlying anatomical structures that may be damaged by massage
c) Areas of major nerves, vessels, arteries, and organs that are exposed
d) All of the above

68. Massage is to be avoided on the popliteal fossa. The endangerment site involved is the:
a) Great saphenous vein
b) Brachiocephelic vein
c) Musculocutaneous nerve
d) None of the above

69. Rolfing is a specialized technique best described as a:
a) Deep connective tissue massage
b) Energy technique
c) Relaxation technique
d) Re-education technique through body movement

70. Kneading (Petrissage) is best described as:
a) The most widely used massage stroke
b) Lifting, grasping, rolling, and compressing
c) Direct pressure on the skin with no gliding
d) Deep, gliding, unidirectional stroke

71. Your client explains they are suffering from a lack of peristalsis. What is the best massage technique to use in this situation?
    a) Gliding strokes which follow the ascending, transverse, & descending colon
    b) Compression over the upper abdomen
    c) Vibration over the lower abdomen
    d) Tapotement over the low back area

72. Select the most desirable stress reduction techniques for a relaxation massage?
    a) Deep breathing and stretching
    b) Meditation and visualization
    c) Deep breathing and active movement
    d) Deep breathing and visualization

73. The benefits of deep transverse friction include:
    a) Broadening of the fibrous muscle tissue
    b) Breaking down fibrous adhesions
    c) Restoring mobility
    d) All of the above

74. Which of the following techniques us the specific movements: "Cradle, Ankle Pull, Leg Press, and Elbow Milk"?
    a) Reiki
    b) NMT
    c) Positional Release
    d) Polarity Therapy

75. Which Acupressure point would you choose for a client who complains of posterior neck and shoulder pain?
    a) ST 36
    b) GB 21
    c) KI 3
    d) LI 4

76. Which channel would you consider using points from to treat a client with symptoms of a common cold including; headache, facial swelling, sore throat, and insomnia?
    a) BL
    b) HT
    c) LI
    d) KI

III - B. ADJUNCT TECHNIQUES AND METHODS

A. Hydrotherapy

1. Definition: **Hydrotherapy** is defined as the use of **water** in any of its three forms (*solid, liquid,* or *vapor*), either internally or externally, in the treatment of disease or trauma. In hydrotherapy, the state of the body is changed by the use of water at varying temperatures applied by a variety of mechanical means. Physiological changes are in direct proportion to the varying environmental changes.

2. Definitions of Importance

Anesthetic - Reduces local pain
Anodyne - Pain reduction
Antipyretic - Reduction in fever
Antispasmodic - Reducing spasms
Chemotaxis - Ability of white blood cells to locate and attack pathogens
Derivation - The drawing of blood to an area (local effects of heat)
Diapedesis - Movement of cells into circulation
Diaphoretic - To increase sweat
Fomentation - Application of moist heat - usually local - to the body surface
Hypnotic - Induces sleep
Purgative – causing vomiting or bowel evacuation
Retrostasis - the drawing of blood to the internal organs
Revulsion - movement or pushing of blood out of an area (local effects of cold)
Sedative - causes CNS to decrease responses of nerve stimuli for relaxation
Stimulant - Increases nerve stimulation.
Tonic - Increases vigor (affusion, ablution, cold shower, or salt glow)

3. Properties of Water

Water has certain particular properties, which render it an excellent therapeutic agent.

> **a.** *Conductor of heat* - Water possesses the ability to absorb and distribute large quantities of heat. Water has 27 times greater capacity for conducting heat than air. It takes only one calorie of heat to raise one gram of water 1 degree C. It is able to give up its heat rapidly, but does not cool too quickly.

> **b.** *Exists in three states - solid, liquid,* and *vapor*, within a relatively narrow range of temperature. As ice, it is effective as a cooling agent; as a liquid, water may be applied by immersion baths, sprays, packs, and douches at any desired temperature and pressure; as a vapor, it may be utilized in steam or vapor baths and by inhalation. (32 degrees F is the

freezing point of water, 98.6 degrees F is human *oral* body temperature, and 212 degrees F is the boiling point of water).

c. *Solvent* - Water can readily dissolve many other substances to form solutions (i.e. electrolytes and sugars).

d. *Inexpensive* - Water is easily accessible and may be applied with relatively inexpensive equipment. It is a universal solvent and non-irritating.

e. *Buoyancy* - Because the density of water is near that of the human body, it produces a buoyant effect upon immersion equal to the weight of the water displaced. Buoyancy can compensate for weakened muscles that are unable to move a heavy limb.

* Also, upon immersion of the body in water, hydrostatic pressure is exerted on the body surface which increases venous and lymph flow from peripheral areas, and can increase urine output.

4. Standards for "Hot" and "Cold"

The terms "hot" and "cold" are relative to body temperature. Ranges above body temperature are warm or hot, and those below body temperature are cool or cold.

Dangerously Hot	**125 degrees F and above**
Painfully Hot	**111 to 124 degrees F**
Very hot	**105 to 110 degrees F**
Hot *	**100 to 104 degrees F**
Warm	**92 to 100 degrees F**
Neutral	**94 to 97 degrees F** (average skin temperature)
Tepid	**80 to 92 degrees F**
Cool	**70 to 80 degrees F**
Cold	**55 to 70 degrees F**
Very Cold	**32 to 55 degrees F**

* One author considers "Hot" to be from 101° to 110° F

The human body maintains a relatively constant temperature despite sizeable variations in environmental temperatures. There are temperature receptors for hot and cold located throughout the body, which transmit impulses to the **hypothalamus**. There, neurons, known as *thermal receptors*, are stimulated by a very slight increase in the temperature of the blood above the point at which the human thermostat is set, normally about 37 degrees C (98.6 degrees F). Whenever the temperature increases by as little as 0.01 above 37 degrees C, these eventually, via sympathetic nerves, reach sweat glands and blood vessels of the skin. They stimulate the body's 2 million or more sweat glands to increase their rates of secretion. The hypothalamus also stimulates the *thyroid gland* to increase cellular metabolism which influences most of the cells of the body. In a cold environment, this homeostatic mechanism works to decrease heat loss and increase heat production.

Together, they almost always succeed in preventing a decrease in blood temperature below the lower limit of normal. Decrease of heat loss results from reduced amounts of sweat secretion and from vasoconstriction of the skin and blood vessels. Increased heat production occurs as a result of shivering and voluntary muscle contractions. Both kinds of muscle work accelerate *catabolism* (the breakdown of molecules into energy), and heat production.

5. Physiological Effects of Hydrotherapy

Physiological changes from hydrotherapy may be classified as **thermal, mechanical,** and **chemical**. Of these effects, thermal is the most important.

    a. *Thermal effects* are produced by the application of water temperatures above or below that of the body. The greater the variation, the greater the physiological effect produced. Heat may be transferred from one object to another, or generated in a substance or tissue, by one of the following methods: *conduction, convection,* or *conversion*.

    In **conduction**, heat is transferred by *direct contact* of one heated object or substance with another. This is the primary manner in which heat is transferred to the body in hydrotherapy. Examples would include: placing of a hot or cold pack to a body surface, and a hot tub bath.

    In **convection**, heat is transferred by moving currents of heated liquids or gases, as in the hot-air furnace or the automobile radiator. Example: heating the air in a sauna to increase body temperature.

    In **conversion**, heat is generated in a substance or tissue by the passage through it of some form of energy. Examples would include: heating of a wire or filament by electricity ; heating of body tissues by diathermy or ultrasound (the conversion of one type of energy to another).

    b. *Mechanical effects* of water upon the body are produced by the *impact* of the water upon the skin surface in whirlpools, sprays, douches, and frictions.

    c. *Chemical effects* of water are produced when it is taken by mouth or when it is used as an irrigation of some body cavity, such as the large bowel. This would also include sitting in an alcohol or Epsom salt bath.

The shifting of fluid from one part of the body to another is known in hydro-therapy as the *hydrostatic effect*. When a large area of the body or the whole body surface is exposed to heat, a general dilation of the blood vessels of the skin takes place. A large quantity of blood is then *shifted* from the interior of the body to the skin. This is the body's method of eliminating heat. It can be used clinically to either send blood to an ischemic area, or remove blood from a hyperemic location.

6. Effects of Heat

The conductive heat of hydrotherapy does not penetrate deeply beneath the skin surface and is confined largely to the skin and subcutaneous tissues. *Moist* heat may penetrate as much a 3.4 centimeters to reach superficial layers of muscle, but is rapidly dissipated by the increased blood flow. Dry heat penetrates less deeply.

    a. *Local* effects of heat
        1) Increase of local circulation and cellular metabolism.
        2) Increase in vasodilation of capillaries, which may be produced by local axon reflexes initiated by stimulation of skin receptors.
        3) Relaxation of skeletal and smooth muscles.
        4) Increased migration of leukocytes through vessel walls in locally heated areas.
        5) Local sweating and local analgesia are produced by moist heat.
        6) Relaxes white connective tissue (dense fibrous).
        7) Contracts yellow connective tissue (layer of fascia under dermis).

    b. *Systemic* effects of heat
        1) Decrease in general metabolism.
        2) Stimulation of nervous system initially, then sedation.
        3) Increase in heart rate (blood in periphery causing the heart to pump faster to fill in the body).
        4) Increases digestion by increasing the release of digestive enzymes.
        5) Increases peristalsis of the stomach, small and large intestine.

General *indications* for the use of heat in hydrotherapy: To relieve cramps and muscle spasms; increase the range of motion of a joint; increase blood flow to areas of poor circulation. Heat is better in the chronic phase of a condition.

General *contra-indications* for the use of heat in hydrotherapy: Acute inflammation, hemorrhage, cancer, decreased sensation or inability to report, and peripheral vascular disease (*often associated with diabetes*).

7. Effects of Cold

Due to the fact that the local application of cold produces vasoconstriction, there is no influx of fresh warm blood to the part. As a result, cold penetrates deeply into the tissues from the surface.

    a. *Local* effects of cold
- **1)** Increase in vasoconstriction.
- **2)** Decrease in local circulation.
- **3)** Decrease in cellular metabolism.
- **4)** Less leukocyte migration through capillary walls.
- **5)** Contraction of skeletal and smooth muscles.
- **6)** Produces a numbing, analgesic, or anesthetic effect (nerve conduction slows).

    b. *Systemic* effects of cold:
- **1)** Stimulation of the nervous system at first, then sedation.
- **2)** Heart rate would first quicken, then decrease.
- **3)** Increase in general metabolism.

General ***indications*** for the use of cold in hydrotherapy: To reduce inflammation (over sprains or strains); acute pain; over trigger points; to increase muscle tone. Cold is better in an acute phase of a condition.

General ***contra-indications*** for the use of cold in hydrotherapy: Cold sensitive or chilled patient, or a patient who cannot report sensations of frostbite.

8. Reflex Effects of Hot and Cold

An adequately intense local application of heat or cold to the skin surface not only affects the immediate skin area, but also other areas in the body via the nervous system. The skin surface carries the stimulus along a nerve fiber to the spinal cord. From there, the stimulus can travel to a related organ or other destination in the body. Generally, the skin area over an organ is in *reflex relationship* to that organ. For example, an ice bag placed over the heart area slows the heart rate and increases its force. A moist, hot pack applied to the skin of the abdomen prior to a meal causes diminished intestinal activity, decreased intestinal blood flow, and decreased gastric acid secretion. The skin segment innervated by a single spinal nerve is known as a ***dermatome***.

    a. *Reflex effects of prolonged heat*
- **1)** Prolonged heat to one extremity causes vasodilation in the contralateral extremity
- **2)** Abdominal wall - Causes decreased intestinal blood flow and diminished intestinal motility; decreases secretion of acid in the stomach

3) Pelvis - Relaxes the musculature of the pelvic organs; dilates the blood vessels, and increases menstrual flow

4) Precordium - Increases the heart rate, decreases its force, and lowers blood pressure

5) Chest - Promotes ease of respiration and expectoration

6) Trunk - Relaxes the ureters or bile ducts; relieves renal or gallbladder colic

7) Kidneys & Lower Abdomen - Increases the production of urine

b. *Reflex effects of prolonged cold*

1) Prolonged cold over the trunk of an artery produces contraction of the artery and its branches

2) Skin over the nose, back of the neck, and hands - Causes contraction of the blood vessels of the nasal mucosa

3) Precordium - Slows the heart rate and increases its stroke volume

4) Abdomen - Increased intestinal blood flow, increased intestinal motility, and increased acid secretion in the stomach

5) Pelvic area - Stimulates the muscles of the pelvic organs

6) Thyroid gland - Contracts its blood vessels and decreases its function

7) Hands and Scalp - Causes contraction of blood vessels to the brain

8) Acutely inflamed joints or bursae - Causes vasoconstriction and relief of pain, and hastens recovery

9) Acute trauma (i.e. contusions, sprains & strains) - Causes vasoconstriction and lessens pain, swelling, and hemorrhage into the tissues

9. Techniques of Local Thermal Procedures

a. *Fomentations:* A local application of *moist heat* to the body surface using a cloth or an electric moist heating pad (*thermophore*).

1) *Effects and Indications*

a) Relief of pain

b) Increase blood flow to an area

c) Relax muscle spasms

d) Produce tissue warming and relaxation in preparation for massage, exercise, electrical stimulation, or ultrasound

e) Promote leukocytosis and diaphoresis

f) Relieve nervous states such as insomnia and nervous tension

g) *Derivation* to increase blood flow peripherally in order to relieve congestion internally

h) Prior to massage

2) Treatment - Cover the part to be treated with a towel(s). Apply fomentation to the area, being aware of the intensity of heat as indicated by the patient's condition and effect to be obtained. The fomentation may be left on the area for 20 to 30 minutes if comfortable to the patient, or changed during treatment.

b. Hydrocollator - *(Aka: Chemical Pack)* Moist heat applied by means of a preheated chemical pack of silica gel. Water is heated to 150 -160 F.

1) *Effects and Indications*
    a) Relieve pain
    b) Increase blood flow to an area
    c) Relax muscle spasm

2) *Treatment* - Place several (6) thicknesses of towel or fomentation cloth over area to be treated. Remove heated pack carefully from hydrocollator and place on the folded towel. Wrap pack with the outer cloth. Leave on area for up to 30 minutes. Dry the skin. Observe that the patient is not perspiring.

c. Paraffin Bath - The local application of melted paraffin to the skin surface.

1) *Effects and Indications*
    a) Hyperemia and other effects of local heat.
    b) Preparation of the skin for massage by making it smooth, soft, and pliable.
    c) For use over: arthritic joints; stiff joints; after fractures or sprains.
    d) For treatment of: bursitis, fibrositis, and tenosynovitis after the acute phase is past.

2) *Treatment* - Wash the part before treatment. Instruct the patient to hold area relaxed in order to avoid cracks in the paraffin. Heat paraffin wax to 122 to 130 degrees F. Dip body part 6 to 12 times, allowing for brief cooling after each dip. Leave paraffin on for 20 to 30 minutes. May wrap part in plastic or cover with a towel to preserve heat. Remove paraffin "glove" and discard.

d. *Hot Foot Bath* - A local immersion bath covering the feet & ankles at temperatures ranging from 100 to 115 degrees F.

1) *Effects and Indications*

   a) Local and reflex effects increase blood flow through the feet and entire skin surface, producing decongestion in the internal organs and brain

   b) Relieve congestive headache, (with cold to the head)

   c) Relieve pelvic congestion

   d) Stop epistaxis (nose bleed)

   e) General warming of the body (to produce sweating when prolonged).

   f) Help prevent or abort a common cold

2) *Treatment* - Have the water 103 degrees F. and deep enough to cover the ankles. Have patient place their feet and ankles in the tub. Add hot water from time to time to increase the temperature to tolerance; ***never*** exceed 115 degrees F. Soak for 10 to 30 minutes.

e. *Whirlpool Bath* - A partial immersion bath in which water is agitated and mixed with air to be directed against the affected area.

1) *Effects and Indications*

   a) Cleanses and stimulates wound healing.

   b) Sedative - Relieves pain and relaxes spasm.

   c) Stimulates circulation.

   d) Softens tissues preparing for massage, stretching, and exercise.

   e) For use on amputation stumps, sprains, and contusions after the first 36 hours, post-operative orthopedic conditions, arthritis and fibrositis, burns, peripheral vascular disease, and peripheral nerve injuries. Use neutral temperatures with vascular disease and neuropathies.

2) *Treatment* - Fill the whirlpool bath to the desired depth at a temperature of 105 to 110 degrees F., or 93 degrees F. Add a tablespoonful of antiseptic to the water. Remove all dressings from patient and seat patient in the bath. Apply a cold compress to the neck and circulate water over areas to be treated. Treatment time is from 10 to 25 minutes.

f. *Sitz Bath* - A partial bath of the pelvic region, given in a special tub.

1) *Effects, Indications, and Time of Treatment*

   a) Hot Sitz (105 to 115 degrees F. for 2 to 10 minutes). Analgesic and stimulant to the pelvic circulation. Indicated in dysmenorrhea, acute and chronic cystitis, chronic pelvic inflammatory disease, prostatitis, and after cystoscopy and hemorrhoidectomy.

b) Cold Sitz (55 to 75 degrees F. for 2 to 10 minutes with friction). Increases the tone of smooth muscle of the uterus, bladder, and colon. Lessens tendency to bleeding from the uterus, lower bowel, and rectum. Indicated in subinvolution of the uterus, metrorrhagia, atonic constipation, and for general tonic effect.

c) Contrast Sitz (Hot phase – 105 to 115 degrees F. for 3 minutes, Cold phase - 55 to 85 degrees F. for 30 seconds). Repeat sequence 3 times. Indicated to increase pelvic circulation and tone of smooth muscle of the pelvic region. For chronic pelvic inflammatory disease, chronic prostatitis, chronic constipation, fistula in ano, and following rectal surgery.

g. *Ice Pack* - A local application of cold over a covered body segment.

    1) *Effects and Indications*
        a) Relief of pain (cold receptors override pain transmission)
        b) Prevention of ecchymosis and swelling.
        c) Decrease of blood flow, local metabolism and inflammation.
        d) For use of an early treatment of sprains, contusions, soft tissue injuries, acute bursitis, acute joint inflammation from rheumatic fever, rheumatoid arthritis, acute infectious arthritis and immediate treatment of burns.

    2) *Treatment* - Apply the ice pack over the covered area for 20-30 minutes, allowing 10 minutes of rest, and then repeat. Observe reaction of the skin to avoid tissue injury.

    R.I.C.E.: Rest, Ice, Compression, & Elevation

h. *Ice Massage* - Deep circular frictions with ice to produce an effect known as hyperstimulation analgesia. The combination of nerve stimulation from friction and cold receptors serve to compete with and decrease pain perception via the "Gate Theory." This allows the muscle to assume its normal, relaxed state.

    1) *Effects and Indications*
        a) Over trigger points
        b) For acute pain
        c) To increase tone in muscle tissue

2) *Treatment* - Deep circular friction with ice over small area (trigger point). Patient usually describes 3 stages including *slight burning, aching* and *numbness*. Treatment is complete when area is numb and blood rushes to the area.

i. *Contrast Local Applications* - The application of alternate heat and cold to a local area. Often used with *chronic* conditions.

1) *Effects and Indications*
    a) An analgesic through acceleration of local circulation
    b) Stimulate healing in local injuries with ecchymosis (contusions).
    c) Relieve muscle stiffness and pain due to trauma or strain (non-acute conditions)
    d) Stimulate healing in wound infections

2) *Treatment* - Cover area to be treated with a towel. Apply the fomentation as hot as can be tolerated for 3 minutes. Remove fomentation and place a towel wrung from ice water directly to the area for 1 minute. Change 3 times. Next, apply a fomentation for 3 minutes. Make at least 3 complete applications. Alternate applications produce both circulatory and thermal reactions. Maximum effects are obtained with short, intense, alternate applications with cold applied about one-third the time of heat, (3 minutes of hot/one minute of cold).

j. *Salt Glow* - The application of rubbing wet salt on the patient's skin.

1) *Effects and Indications*
    a) Tonic and stimulating
    b) Produces vigorous stimulation of the peripheral circulation
    c) Builds up resistance as a stimulant for persons who do not react well to cold

2) *Treatment* - Wet patient's skin with water. Take both hands full of moistened salt and apply to an extremity and give friction to tolerance. Start with the extremities - then do the chest, back, and buttocks. Wash off all salt and dry patient thoroughly. Note that the salt glow should not be given if there is infective skin disease present.

k. Alcohol Rub - Application of rubbing alcohol to surface of the body

1) *Effects and Indications*
    a) Lower body temperature in fevers

      b) Cooling effect after general or local applications of heat

      c) Protects pressure areas by astringent effect on the skin

      d) Refresh the patient when a bath is not given

2) *Treatment* - Use rubbing alcohol or 95% pure grain alcohol diluted to make a 70% solution (alcohol 2/3 to water 1/3). Pour alcohol into cupped hands. Rub upper extremities first with upward strokes. For cooling effects, use short alternating strokes to aid evaporation of the alcohol. Apply to chest, lower extremities, and back.

l. *Hubbard Tank* - A specially constructed, full-immersion tub with a turbine for administering underwater exercises, using neutral or mild heat.

1) *Effects and Indications*

      a) Relaxing and cleansing

      b) Aids in exercise and stretching

      c) Increases circulatory effects and aids in mobilization (Saline and brine solutions aid in treatment of burns and decubitus ulcers)

      d) Used in treatment for rheumatoid arthritis, neuromuscular conditions (multiple sclerosis, cerebral palsy, Parkinson's Disease, hemiplegia, poliomyelitis), post-operative orthopedic conditions, burns, and decubitus ulcers.

2) *Treatment* - Water temperature should be between 90 and 100 degrees F. Assist patient into the tank. The turbine may be directed to specific areas for a hydro massage effect. After a warming period or application of the turbine, stretching procedures, range-of-motion exercises, passive and/or active, may proceed. Time: 20 to 30 minutes. Assist patient from the tank, dry thoroughly, and have patient rest after treatment.

m. *Russian Bath* - A body steam bath given while the patient reclines with the head outside of the steam cabinet (head not exposed to the heat).

1) *Effects and Indications*

      a) Increase body temperature (no heat loss because of 100% humidity).

      b) Production of a short, mild fever with sweating.

      c) Increase in pulse rate, blood pressure, and metabolism.

      d) Increase in peripheral vasodilation.

      e) Indicated for rheumatoid arthritis, gout, obesity, alcoholism, and other addictions.

2) *Treatment* - Temperature in the steam room should be 110 to 120 degrees F. Assist patient into the steam room, having them lie horizontally on his back, with the head outside the room. Place a cold compress around the neck, and apply an ice bag to the heart if the pulse is 80 or above. Turn the steam on gradually. Time: 5 to 10 minutes. Take the patient's pulse every 5 minutes and give water to drink as necessary. Stay with the patient. Assist patient out of steam room and have him rest after treatment. This procedure is *contraindicated* in: hypertension; diabetes; cardiac impairment; disorders which include diminished circulatory capability, or decreased sensitivity.

n. *Brand Bath* - A cold immersion bath with friction.

1) *Effects and Indications*
    a) Fever reduction
    b) Excite immune system

2) *Treatment* - Assist the patient into a tub of water at 60 to 70 degrees F. Use a sponge to the body surface and rub vigorously for 2 to 3 minutes. Have patient sit up and pour cold water over the head. The patient lies back again and rubs vigorously for 5 minutes. Continue the alternate rubbing and cold water pouring for 10 to 20 minutes.

o. *Neutral Bath* - Immersion of the body in a tub of water at a neutral temperature (94 to 98 degrees F).

1) *Effects and Indications*
    a) Use as a sedative for central nervous exhaustion
    b) Help alleviate insomnia
    c) Decrease nervous irritability
    (The sedative effect is a response to neutral temperature not being stimulating to the body and the water prevents external skin stimuli.)

2) *Treatment* - Assist the patient into the tub, placing a pillow or towel under the head. Ask the patient to lie quietly and relax. Stay with the patient. Duration of the bath can be 15 to 20 minutes, or up to 3 or 4 hours (add warm water to maintain the temperature). Assist patient out of the tub and dry gently. The patient should have undisturbed rest for at least 30 minutes following a neutral bath.

B. Heliotherapy

Heliotherapy is defined as the treatment of a patient by exposure to a form of *light*. Light sources used in heliotherapy include: *electric, ultraviolet,* and *infrared*.

1. Electric Light Bath - An application of heat to the body by radiant energy from the use of incandescent light bulbs. May use a small, hand-held lamp for local application, or an electric light cabinet for general application.

    a. *Effects and Indications*
- 1) To reduce blood pressure due to marked peripheral vasodilation.
- 2) To produce sweating and a slight increase in temperature.
- 3) Mild heating for: neuroses, rheumatic conditions, chronic nephritis, peripheral neuritis, psychoneurosis, obesity, and hypertensive vascular disease.

    b. *Treatment* - Hold incandescent light over area to be treated for 5 to 8 minutes, or have patient sit in the cabinet with the lights on for 5 to 8 minutes. Do not touch the lights. Have patient rest after treatment. *Contraindicated* if the patient has: diabetes, cardiac impairment, advanced arteriosclerosis, or if patient is emaciated.

2. Ultraviolet Light Therapy - A local application of a specific (UV) frequency of light to the body or a body segment by energy from an ultraviolet light source.

    a. *Effects and Indications*
- 1) Antiseptic
- 2) Sterilize an area
- 3) Treatment for acne, psoriasis, and fungal infections

    b. *Treatment* - Hold the ultraviolet source approximately 2 to 3 feet from area being treated. The first treatment of the area is for a period of 30 seconds, second treatment for 60 seconds and third treatment for 90 seconds with a period of 24 hours between *each* treatment. General *contra-indications* would include: hypersensivity to light, cancer, open bleeding, and pus.

3. Infrared Light Therapy - A local treatment of heat to a body segment with the use of vibrating infrared (IR) light rays.

    a. *Effects and Indications* - (Same indications as hot packs)
- 1) Relaxation
- 2) Reduce muscle spasms and pain from arthritis and cramps
- 3) Increase range of motion of a joint
- 4) Prior to massage

      b. *Treatment* - Infrared light source is held 1 to 2 feet away from area being treated. The length of treatment is 20-30 minutes. General ***contra-indications*** would include decreased sensitivity in limbs and acute traumatic injuries.

C. Exercise & Stress Reduction

Exercise, breathing techniques, relaxation techniques, and stress management techniques are recognized by some as alternative ways to reduce pain and anxiety. Kabat-Zinn, molecular biologist and assistant professor of medicine at the Massachusetts Medical Center, founded their stress reduction clinic, which has been a model for other centers. He states that because the word "meditation" may have negative connotations for some people, he uses the term "Mindfulness". He teaches his patient's to live in the moment. He teaches them to "scan" their bodies, move through the pain, and relax into their discomfort." He teaches Yoga techniques stating that if the patient can change their body language and physical posture, they can change their attitudes and feelings.

Biofeedback techniques can help people cope with pain. Dr. Karen Olness, M.D. and Professor of Pediatrics, Family Medicine and International Health at Case Western Reserve University, demonstrated how children learned to cope with migraine headaches and reduce the number of attacks through biofeedback. The children recognized through computer images when their minds were relaxed and could regulate the frequency and severity of these headaches. Dr. Olness defines the differences between some techniques; she states, "Meditation's purpose is going within and quieting." Self-hypnosis or relaxation imagery is for a specific purpose--often relieving pain.

However, Dr. Olness and Herbert Benson, Professor of medicine at Harvard, think there is no difference in the state, just in the purpose. Mr. Benson's study could not differentiate between body temperature, heart rate, pulse, or brain wave patterns in any of these states. According to Dr. Olness, there are encouraging studies being conducted in this area, but are to date inconclusive. She feels these techniques allow an individual to take control of one's thinking and in turn, feel they have control over their body's response.

John Zawacki, M.D., Director of Clinical Services in the Division of Digestive Disease and Nutrition, University of Massachusetts Medical Center, uses various stress reduction techniques with his patients. The results usually show changes including:
      1. **Adaptation** - The patient realizes that he or she can carry on in their daily lives despite pain.
      2. **Improvement** - Better able to deal with their pain in ways that do not interfere with daily life.
      3. **Coping** – Patient requires fewer visits, less medication, and is happier overall.

David Spiegel, M.D., Professor of Psychiatry and Behavioral Sciences and Director of the Psychosocial Treatment Laboratory, Stanford University School of Medicine, completed a study of women with metastatic breast cancer. The group of women could not change the fact they were dying, but could take control of their mental states, alleviating some of the helplessness they were feeling.

Erik Pepper, Ph.D., San Francisco State University, Vietta S. Wilson, Ph.D. York University and Will Taylor, M.D., conclude that repetitive strain injury (i.e. chronic neck or upper limb pain) in computer users can be prevented by:

1. Proper ergonomics (work station configuration).
2. Work pattern variation (work/rest cycles).
3. Self-regulation through biofeedback to reduce muscle bracing.
4. Relaxation/strengthening practices (progressive relaxation & physiological quieting are two methods).
5. Emotional Control - develop communication/problem solving skills.

He states that ***kinesthetic awareness*** and the ***skills to reduce tension*** are necessary for any change. Changing the configuration of a workstation etc. and work patterns are not enough. In their study, surface EMG monitoring provided feedback when muscles began to tense during daily activities, allowing for proper adjustments, exercise, relaxation techniques, etc.

REVIEW QUESTIONS - ADJUNCT TECHNIQUES AND METHODS

1. The movement of fluid from tissues in one part of the body to tissues in another area of the body is known as:
    a) Chemotaxis
    b) Hydrostatic Effect
    c) Conversion
    d) Thermal Effect

2. When using a Chemical Pack (Hydrocollator), the water temperature in the tank should be approximately:
    a) 125 - 135 F.
    b) 140 - 180 F.
    c) 150 - 160 F.
    d) 105 - 115 F.

3. One of the more common conditions for which a massage therapist might use the Paraffin Bath is:
    a) Acute Sprains and Strains
    b) Rheumatoid Arthritis
    c) Swelling
    d) Malignant Melanoma

4. The most beneficial use of alternate hot/cold (contrast) treatments is with:
    a) Acute muscle spasm
    b) Chronic muscle spasm
    c) Insulin dependent diabetes
    d) Acute Fibromyalgia

5. Alternative methods of stress reduction & relaxation techniques include:
    a) Breathing techniques
    b) Visualization
    c) Biofeedback
    d) All of the above

6. The name given in hydrotherapy to a local application of moist heat is:
    a) Steam Bath
    b) Infusion
    c) Fomentation
    d) Vaso Pack

7. Circle the *incorrect* statement regarding alternative ways to reduce pain & stress.
    a) Meditation's purpose is to go within and quiet.
    b) Relaxation imagery does not contribute to stress or pain reduction.
    c) Techniques that manage pain include having clients scan their body, moving through the pain, & relaxing into their discomfort.
    d) Yoga can change a client's body language & physical posture, which in turn can change attitudes & feelings.

8. Which of the following is *not* indicated as form of treatment for an acute sprain or strain:
    a) Ice
    b) Elevation
    c) Compression
    d) Fomentation

9. Which of the following is *not* an indication for the hot Whirlpool Bath:
    a) Peripheral nerve damage
    b) Rheumatoid arthritis
    c) Non-acute sprains/strains
    d) Prior to massage

10. Joint mobility and range of motion are increased by which of the following:
    a) Hydrocollator packs
    b) Hot whirlpool bath
    c) Russian bath
    d) All of the above

11. Contraindications for heat therapy would include all of the following *except*:
    a) Cancer
    b) Diabetes
    c) Edema
    d) Spastic colon

12. Heat treatments for diabetic patients are contraindicated because of:
    a) Increased local cell metabolism
    b) Decreased nervous system function
    c) Decreased arterial function
    d) All of the above

13. Hyperstimulation of cold and pressure receptors as explained by the Gate Theory in the treatment of muscle spasms, is best facilitated by the use of the following therapy:
    a) Hydrocollator pack
    b) Neutral baths
    c) Contrast baths
    d) Ice massage

14. Which of the following is *not* a general contraindication for hydrotherapy?
    a) Diabetes
    b) Acute trauma
    c) Cancer
    d) Congestive heart failure

15. The application of moist heat is superior to that of dry heat because of:
    a) Convection
    b) Conduction
    c) Conversion
    d) The Greenhouse Effect

16. The Hubbard Tank is used to administer underwater exercises with the use of:
    a) Very cold water
    b) Alcohol rub
    c) Steam
    d) Neutral or mild heat

17. Which is true regarding the local effect of cold therapy?
    a) Vasodilation
    b) Increases circulation
    c) Vaso constriction
    d) Increases local metabolism

18. Which treatment would be used for a patient diagnosed with Multiple Sclerosis?
    a) Hot sitz bath
    b) Hot whirlpool bath
    c) Neutral whirlpool
    d) Cold packs

19. Which treatment would you use prior to massage with your patient who has Fibromyalgia?
    a) Cold packs
    b) Hydrocollator
    c) Neutral bath
    d) Contrast hot/cold

20. What effect would systemic heat treatments have on a patient with diabetes?
    a) Increase blood sugar
    b) Cause hemorrhage
    c) Decrease blood sugar
    d) No effect

IV. BUSINESS PRACTICES, PROFESSIONAL STANDARDS, & ETHICS

Business practices and professionalism are a necessary and important part of an LMT's training. LMTs must abide by high ethical standards to uphold the acceptance of their profession in the health care field and overcome the public's negative image (massage parlors), as well as provide the best care possible for their clients. Training in basic First Aid/CPR is required to protect the client's health, safety, and welfare so one can properly respond in an emergency.

A. Business Practices

1. Business Plan
Formulating a comprehensive business plan increases your chances of success. A typical business plan will usually include the following items:

   a. Cover Page: Title, name, address, & telephone.
   b. Table of Contents - Listing business plan sections & page numbers
   c. Owners Statement - Description of business & the owner.
   d. Executive Summary - Business plan highlights.
   e. Purpose & Goals - Business (career) goals & priorities.
   f. Detailed Business Description - History & mission statement.
   g. Marketing Plan - Promotion, Advertising, Publicity, P/R, & budget
   h. Risk Assessment - Competition, industry trends, & contingency.
   i. Financial Analysis - Personal & business financial statements.
   j. Operations - Organizational policies & procedures.
   k. Success Strategies - Plans, flow charts, support systems, etc.
   l. Appendix - Additional supporting information & documents.

2. Professional Image
The professional image is an outward reflection of a therapist's personal presentation, office presentation, and general business practices. Items that contribute to this image are dress, communication skills, phone skills, call-back punctuality, personal hygiene, appointment punctuality, community involvement, office location, neatness & cleanliness, displays of professional licenses & certifications, business cards & brochures, clinical skills, empathy & understanding, respect of confidentiality, and appropriate referral policy.

3. Business, Accounting Practices, & Taxes
Each type of business entity has specific tax and liability advantages and disadvantages. Sole proprietorships, partnerships, and corporations are the most common forms of businesses. In most cases it is paramount to seek the advice of a CPA before deciding which type of business structure is best for you. A massage practice dictates that there be two types of records prepared. These are business or financial records and client or medical records.

a. Knowledge of basic business principals is necessary to keep accurate records and report your income correctly on your Federal income tax return. It is very important to seek professional assistance in the areas of record keeping, good accounting practices, proper reporting of income (*all compensation*, whether money or barter), payment of taxes, and employment status (employee vs. independent contractor). You may wish to form a corporation because it limits *personal* liability for the business debts. However, there are specific legal requirements, as well as more complicated record keeping issues, which are not covered in this review. Lack of knowledge may result in audits by the IRS.

b. Employment status: Employee or independent contractor? The IRS uses strict guidelines to determine if an individual is an employee or independent contractor (self-employed). For example: If you work for a chiropractor and he/she provides the clients, schedules the appointments, provides the table, space & supplies, handles all the insurance billing, and the client pays the chiropractor directly for the massage, you would usually be considered an employee. Your employer is responsible for withholding income and social security tax from your wages. He/she also contributes a portion toward your social security tax. You are issued a Form W-2 for reporting your income taxes. Business expenses are limited, and you need to check the rules and regulations on any business expense you are entitled to deduct.

However, if you *contract* with an individual or company to provide massage services for a percentage of the fee, you **may** be considered an independent contractor and self-employed. A *written contract* should be made; it is very important to consult with a professional before signing a contract to make sure that the employment status is being handled correctly. As an independent contractor, you are issued a Form 1099 to report income taxes. Nothing is withheld from the pay, and you are responsible for paying the income and social security taxes. In this instance, the payer does not contribute anything toward your social security tax, and you pay a higher percentage than if you were an employee (see IRS regulations for portion you can deduct). You are entitled to certain business expense deductions, and the income and expenses are reported on Schedule C of your income tax return.

The same is true if you are a sole proprietor of a business or form a partnership; you are considered self-employed. You are paid directly by the client. The total income and business expenses are reported on special schedules with the income tax return, and again you are responsible for your own taxes. As a sole proprietor, you file a Schedule C with the income tax return. If you form a partnership, each partner shares in the income and expenses of the business. The partnership must file a Form l065, Federal Partnership Tax Return, reporting the gross income, and deductible business expenses. Each partner receives a Schedule K-1, showing their portion of the net income or loss for the year, and this schedule is filed with their individual income tax return.

If one is self-employed, he is required to file an estimated tax return, Form l040ES, **quarterly** with the IRS and pay any tax that is due. Because he is self-employed, quarterly payments are required, based on your estimated tax liability. Failure to do so can result in an estimated tax penalty plus interest.

Regardless of business structure, one may choose to obtain a Federal Tax Identification Number or EIN. This number is used for all state or federal reporting and for opening of business bank accounts (instead of your social security number). Use the IRS form SS-4 to apply for an EIN.

4. Insurance

There are several different types of insurance coverage available to protect the LMT, establishment owner, landlord, and client.

a. *Property Damage and Bodily Injury Liability insurance* is coverage that pays the client if they are injured from an accident while on the establishment site (trip, slip, and fall, or injury due to equipment failure). This insurance may be required by a landlord or employer to reduce their liability. Some state laws require this type of insurance for "establishments."

b. *Malpractice insurance* is generally not required by law, but protects a LMT and pays the client who has successfully sued a LMT for injuries/damages suffered as a result of the massage. Professional organizations and insurance agents can give advice regarding what kind of insurance you need and the suggested coverage limits.

c. *Business & Personal Property Loss insurance* reimburses the owner for loss due to fire, water damage, or theft of business or personal equipment. Homeowners insurance may apply in some circumstances.

d. *Disability insurance* pays the therapist if he/she is unable to work because of an illness, injury, or other covered condition.

      e. ***Automobile insurance*** may have to be upgraded if an auto is used for business purposes.

5. Licensure

Various state, county, and/or city licenses or permits may be necessary. Most cities and/or counties require a business or *occupational* license. This may require that a business location meet appropriate zoning and health department requirements. Some cities and counties require occupational licenses for "mobile" therapists. Many states have licensure requirements for massage therapists. Check with individual states for educational, testing, and licensure requirements. Some cities and/or counties may require certification (usually in lieu of state licensure). Some states require that the massage office or *establishment* be licensed. Check with state and local agencies for specific details. If you sell products to your clients, you may be required to obtain additional licensure and a state *sales tax permit*. Additional requirements may include monthly or quarterly reporting with payment of taxes collected.

B. Professional Standards

As members of the health care industry, it is extremely important to project a professional and caring image.

1. Professional Boundaries dictate the *limits of interaction* between persons.

Personal boundaries include the physical, emotional, and privacy limits that a therapist might establish to protect themselves. The act of writing down one's boundaries helps to explore and clarify them. Establishing and maintaining personal boundaries may preserve one's physical and emotional health. Professional boundaries are generally client-focused and help to define the therapist-client relationship. They generally include limits with regard to physical touch, pain, nudity, intimacy, social interaction, remuneration, gift giving, confidentiality, and appropriateness of sharing personal (non-massage related) information. Inherent in the client / therapist relationship is the potential for transference and counter-transference. *Transference* means that feelings (positive or negative) that a client has for a significant person in their (early) life are unconsciously transferred to the therapist. *Countertransference* is the unconscious emotional reaction of the therapist to the client, based upon the therapist's inner (positive or negative) desires and needs. Maintaining professional and personal boundaries may help to limit both transference and counter-transference. Termination of the therapeutic relationship may be necessary if boundaries are not maintained.

2. Interviewing Techniques

Several interviewing models exist for obtaining the data necessary to initiate (and continue) the therapeutic relationship. All interview models stress the establishment of a *trust-based relationship* and "*active listening*". Affirm the confidential nature of your client's information. The medical history provides a jumping-off-point for further information gathering. Information is available from the client in both verbal and non-verbal form. Questions should be open-ended and objective. "Artful phrasing" encourages a response. Non-threatening information should be gathered first. Eye contact and non-verbal cues encourage trust and sharing. Explain why you need the information. Gather as much detail about the complaints as possible. Summarize the information you have gathered and confirm your findings. Thank the client for sharing the information with you. Proceed to the "hands-on interview" (examination) where you continue to observe and listen, as you palpate and test. Share your assessment with the client and discuss treatment strategy options.

3. Communication Skills

Communication can be verbal, non-verbal, or written. First impressions set the tone for future communication. Verbal communication is facilitated by a trusting relationship or rapport. Speak clearly, slowly, simply, directly, and honestly. Ask questions and *listen*. Make eye contact and give non-verbal acknowledgement. Reflective feedback lets the other person(s) know that you are listening. Written communication should be word-processed on professional letterhead. Use the proper title (Dr., Mr., Mrs., Ms., etc.) and last name. Be clear, specific, and concise. Summarize details. Use language appropriate to the situation, (medical terminology is appropriate for health care professionals, but may not be, for the potential client who inquires about your practice). Enclose copies when appropriate. Common examples of written communication are: Introductory Letters, Initial Reports, SOAP Charts, Progress Reports, Discharge Reports, and Letters of Referral.

4. Client Record Keeping or Charting

Informed Consent refers specifically to having the client acknowledge, in writing, the agreed upon therapeutic goals, procedures, and their rationales.

HIPAA, the Health Insurance Portability and Accountability Act is a federal standard designed to protect the medical records of individuals. The HIPAA Privacy Rule is administered by the U.S. Dept. of Health and Human Services. This act states that records must be kept secure, (locked and inaccessible) yet be made available to clients upon request.

S.O.A.P. charting refers to the standard system for recoding medical data. The SOAP chart documents the client's health information and goals, the therapist's findings and treatment, the client's response to therapy, and the progress toward goals. The "S" refers to *subjective* - data provided by the client. The "O" refers to *objective* - findings of the therapist. These might include observation of signs, palpatory findings, ROM in degrees, or results of specialized tests. The "A" refers to *assessment* - functional outcomes or findings (diagnosis in medical practice). The "P" refers to *plan* - treatment recommendations. Documentation should contribute to the therapeutic process. Chart only information that is pertinent to the client's case. Record information in a factual manner. Make assessments based upon factual data. Ensure that treatment goals will lead to positive functional outcomes by making them specific, measurable, attainable, relevant, and time-sensitive. Use terminology consistent with the medical standard for record keeping, including common medical abbreviations. Initial notes, subsequent notes, progress notes, and discharge notes should be consistent. Discharge notes should summarize treatment dates (including those missed or canceled), current health status, progress summary, reason for termination of care, recommendations for ongoing care, and referrals made.

5. Third Party Reimbursement

Massage therapists in some states are eligible to directly bill and collect payment for services from third party payers. These payers may include Commercial Health Insurance carriers (Med Pay), Managed Care Plans (HMOs, PPOs), Workers Compensation carriers, Auto Insurance carriers (PIP), State Insurers (uninsured motorists, etc.), and Federal Healthcare programs (Medicare & Medicaid). When a massage therapist is eligible for direct payment, several criteria must be met. The client (patient) must have a medical diagnosis (with an appropriate ICD-10 diagnostic code). There must, in most cases, be a written prescription for massage therapy. Medial necessity for the massage therapy may have to be established. Billing must be done on standard billing forms (HCFA 1500) using the appropriate (CPT) procedural codes. Proper documentation and timely submission of forms are imperative. Therapists who wish to pursue third party reimbursement may want to enlist the aid of a professional billing service. These businesses usually charge a minimal fee for this very tedious and specialized service. When a licensed physician *employs* a massage therapist, the burden of collection falls upon the physician.

6. Confidentiality

Confidentiality is an ethical principal based upon the clients right to privacy. HIPAA, the Health Insurance Portability and Accountability Act, was enacted in 1996, and requires health care providers to protect the health care records of individuals. Therapists must inform clients about their privacy rights and how their health care information will be used. Confidentiality is a legal matter and information shared with a therapist cannot be divulged, except in certain conditions, such as when consulting with other health care professionals, clinical supervisors, or if required by law. Professional associations and certification boards have established specific guidelines for confidentiality issues and the massage profession.

7. Health Care Professionals: Communication & Referral
Understanding the role of other health care professionals, communication, and making appropriate referrals are a critical element in projecting a professional image. When needed, appropriate *referral to other LMTs with specialized training or to other health care providers is* an ethical duty. Below is a list of various health care professionals and a brief description of their roles:

a. Chiropractic Physician - Uses system of manipulations and treatment to the structures of the body, especially the spinal column, based on the theory that disease is caused by abnormal function of the nervous system.

b. Dermatologist - Physician specializing in disorders of the skin.

c. Endocrinologist - Physician specializing in the endocrine system.

d. Licensed Acupuncturist - Graduate of an approved acupuncture school who has completed state requirements for licensure. Licensed acupuncturists have training in traditional Chinese medicine as well as Chinese herbs, acupuncture, electroacupuncture and tui na.

e. Naturopathic Physician - Graduate of a four-year residential medical school, with training in standard medical sciences, botanical medicine, hydrotherapy, physiotherapy, nutrition, homeopathy, and manipulation. May employ X-ray, laboratory diagnosis, and allopathic pharmaceuticals.

f. Occupational Therapist - Utilizes therapeutic use of work, self-care, and play activities to increase independent function, enhance development, prevent disability, and increase quality of life.

g. Orthopedist - Surgeon specializing in techniques pertaining to the correction of deformities of the musculoskeletal system.

h. Osteopathic Physician - Utilizes generally accepted physical, medicinal, and surgical methods of diagnosis and therapy, while placing chief emphasis on the importance of normal body mechanics, interrelationship of the musculoskeletal system to other body systems, and manipulative methods of detecting and correcting faulty structures.

i. Physical Therapist - Utilizes massage, manipulation, therapeutic exercise, hydrotherapy, etc. to assist in rehabilitation and restoration of normal bodily function after illness or injury.

j. Podiatrist - Physician trained in the examination, diagnosis, and treatment of abnormal nails, and superficial growths occurring on the feet, including corns, warts, callous, bunions, and arch troubles with medical, surgical, mechanical, and physiotherapy treatment.

k. Psychiatrist - Physician specializing in the study, diagnosis, and treatment of mental diseases.

l. Psychologist - Person trained to perform psychological examinations, therapy, and research on the mind, especially behavioral manifestations.

C. Ethics

Many state and national massage and bodywork associations have their own code for ethical and professional behavior. Following is a summary of these ethical guidelines:

1. When needed, refer your client to another LMT certified in special modalities; i.e. Myofascial, Lymphatic, NMT, Cranio-Sacral, Trager, Rolfing, etc. These specialized treatments require advanced training. Attempting to use these treatments without the proper training is unethical and could harm the client.

2. Understand the physiological effects massage and other bodywork modalities have on the body and the possible precautions/contraindications. Obtain a physician's recommendation when appropriate. If in doubt, do not massage that day. Research, consult with his/her physician (with client's permission), etc. and reschedule the massage. If massage is contraindicated, do not massage. Explain why and refer to other health care professionals if appropriate.

3. Do not perform any service *outside* the scope of your practice. Provide treatment only when there is reasonable expectation it can help your client. Respect your client's choices in traditional health care. When needed, refer the client to the appropriate health care provider; i.e. chiropractor, M.D., physical therapist, psychotherapist, etc.

4. Educate your clients about the benefits of massage and their responsibilities; i.e. how and why massage works, stretching techniques, etc.

5. Make no false claims about the benefits of massage.

6. Maintain open, honest, and confidential communication with your client. Be sensitive to and respect your client's wishes and pain tolerance. Keep clear and accurate written documentation (in-take forms and progress notes). Accurate notes are a vital part of your treatment plan. (These notes may also be used in litigation for insurance claims or a mal-practice suit.)

7. Respect the client's boundaries. Provide proper draping. Understand their individual right to privacy, emotional expression, and beliefs.

8. Honest advertising--do not advertise specialized techniques or treatments unless you have the proper training.

9. Project a professional image for yourself, your business, and your profession. Dress in accordance with what is accepted as suitable for business and professional practice.

10. Do not practice under the influence of alcohol or drugs.

11. Be aware and do not tolerate sexual advances. Avoid suggestive advertising.

12. Membership in professional associations broadens your knowledge and keeps you informed about important legislation/trends in the profession as well as educational articles. Advance your education and strive to expand your knowledge and competency.

13. Refuse any gift in excess of what is accepted practice, which may be intended to influence a referral, treatment, etc.

14. Provide Fee Schedule to Client. Professionals set their fees based on the cost of doing business, market place, and level of service provided. According to the FSMTA, fees for prescribed work are usually higher than non-prescribed work. Fee schedules can avoid unpleasant, unnecessary, and costly misunderstandings.

15. Abide by all State and local regulations.

V. FIRST AID & CPR

This review is intended only as an outline of the information presented by the American Red Cross's, *Community First Aid and Safety, 2002 Edition,* which is used as a training manual for introductory first aid and CPR courses.

HIV, hepatitis, and other pathogens are commonly transmitted by exposure to blood and other body fluids. Always use "*universal precautions*" when administering first aid. Please refer to above-mentioned text for complete details of First Aid/CPR procedures.

Injuries (including accidents, suicides and homicides) rank fourth as the leading cause of death among Americans, preceded by heart disease, cancer, and strokes. Each year more than 140,000 Americans die from injuries. Among Americans under the age of 65, injuries rank as the #1 killer.

1. **Definition** - First aid is the immediate care given to the injured or suddenly ill person. This treatment *should not* take the place of proper medical treatment and consists only of furnishing *temporary* assistance until medical care (if needed) arrives. First aid can save a life or aid in the recovery of an injury.

2. **Your Responsibility** - You are required to give first aid only if your job description gives you that responsibility or you have a pre-existing responsibility to another person (client/therapist).

Once you begin to give first aid you must continue until relieved by a medical professional or another qualified first aid caregiver. You must provide the *"level of care"* expected of a reasonable person who has the same level of training you do. This standard of care must follow published recommended first aid procedures (American Heart Association, etc.).

You must attempt to gain the injured person's consent (or that of a parent/guardian). If the injured person is unconscious, you should give care, as it is understood that you have "*implied consent.*" Injured persons have the right to refuse care and that decision must be honored. Although you are generally safe from liability when acting under *good faith* and *within* the limits of your training, an injured party can sue you.

3. **Assessment of the Injured Person** - The goal of any victim assessment is to gain the victim's consent and confidence, and to gather information relating to their injuries and medical condition. The assessment is completed in two steps-- the primary and secondary survey.

The ***primary survey*** includes assessment of the victim's immediate condition and relates to the following areas: (1) **A**irway, (2) **B**reathing, (3) **C**irculation, (4) Hemorrhage, hereafter referred to the **ABC's of First Aid.** Remember to address any problems before going to the secondary survey.

The *secondary survey* is a systematic head-to-toe examination of the victim, looking for abnormalities of the various systems. Assessing the signs and symptoms presented may reveal non-life threatening problems.
*Note: a medical alert tag may give you information about a specific condition the victim might have. Look for important signs and symptoms of injury. Start by looking at the victim's head, then neck, trunk, and extremities for abnormalities such as swelling, tenderness, and discoloration which might indicate an unseen injury.

4. Obtain Emergency Medical Support - Summon medical assistance by **calling 911** or other local community emergency number. Give the following information over the telephone: **Victim's location** with landmarks; phone number you are calling from; nature of the emergency; how many people need help & any special circumstances; condition of victim(s) & what is being done for the victim(s). *Always speak slowly and clearly, and be the last one to hang up the phone.

5. Basic Life Support - CPR - Cardiopulmonary Resuscitation combines rescue breathing (mouth to mouth) and external chest compressions. CPR can save lives in cases of heart attack, drowning, suffocation, electrocution, and drug overdose. *Use CPR any time a victim's breathing and heart have stopped (use rescue breathing alone if there is a pulse but no breathing).

    a. *Procedure* - Call for Emergency Medical Services **first** (911), then begin CPR. Most victims needing CPR will not survive unless they receive advanced cardiac life support services (defibrillation, oxygen, and drug therapy) within eight minutes. Do not begin CPR if signs of death are present, the victim has been in cardiac arrest for more than 30 minutes (except cold water drowning victims), the victim is in an unsafe environment or when a "do not resuscitate" order is in effect. Cease CPR when the victim regains pulse and breathing; when you are replaced by another trained rescuer (EMS); when you are too exhausted to continue; when the scene becomes unsafe; when directed by physician; or when cardiac arrest lasts more then 30 minutes.

    b. *Complications* of CPR commonly include:
      1) Vomiting - turn victim on side & clear mouth.
      2) Stomach distention - caused by air in stomach. Slow down rescue breathing and use mouth to nose method, insuring airway is open.
      3) Aspiration or inhalation of foreign substances - place victim on their left side.
      4) Chest compression injuries such as rib and sternal fractures, and bruised or lacerated lungs - use proper hand position with smooth compressions.

c. *Basic CPR Steps Include*:

R - Responsiveness
A - Actuate EMS System
P - Position victim on back
A - Airway Open? (head tilt/chin lift)
B - Breathing (look, listen, feel)
B - Breaths (give two)
C - Circulation at Carotid?
C - Chest compressions (15:2) adult - *with children, try to get help (shout) after establishing unresponsiveness, but initiate CPR immediately (send someone else to call for EMS).

6. Foreign Body Airway Obstruction - Choking results in over 3,000 deaths/year. Procedure is as follows: Ask if they are choking?

a. If person is conscious and cannot speak, breath, or cough - Ask if you can help them. Have someone call 911. Give up to five (5) abdominal thrusts **(*Heimlich Maneuver*)**.

b. After each five thrusts, check victim and your technique.

c. Repeat cycles of five thrusts until victim coughs up object, begins to breath or cough forcefully, becomes unconscious, or you are relieved by another trained person.

d. If victim is *unconscious*, It is more important to get air in than to get the object out. Roll victim onto their back and check for breathing, If air is circulating, check for pulse and begin CPR is there is no circulation. If airway is obstructed *perform finger sweep* to remove foreign objects from *mouth*. If your attempts are unsuccessful, give two rescue breaths, then finger sweep - repeat until object is expelled or EMS arrives.

e. In cases of infant choking, use five back blows followed by five chest thrusts. Give two slow breaths between each cycle for unconscious infant. Repeat process until object is expelled or EMS arrives.

7. Shock - A sudden disturbance of mental equilibrium, occurring with an acute failure of the peripheral circulatory system. The following are the most common types of shock:

a. *Hypovolemic Shock* - Results from blood or fluid loss (also known as hemorrhagic shock).

1) Signs and symptoms might include -
a) Pale/bluish skin, nail beds, or lips.

      b) Ashen, cool, moist skin.

      c) Rapid breathing and pulse.

      d) Dilated pupils/sunken look of eyes.

      e) Restlessness or irritability.

      f) Thirst or nausea and vomiting.

      g) Loss of consciousness.

2) First aid for hypovolemic shock includes the following steps -

      a) Have victim lie down - make them comfortable.

      b) Call 911 or local EMS.

      c) Control any external bleeding.

      d) Elevate legs 12 inches (if no spinal, hip, or leg injury).

      e) Maintain body heat.

      f) Reassure the victim.

b. *Fainting* - Described as a sudden, temporary loss of consciousness. It occurs when the brain's blood supply is interrupted.

1) Fainting may be preceded or accompanied by -

      a) Dizziness

      b) Seeing spots

      c) Nausea

      d) Paleness

      e) Sweating

2) First aid for fainting includes -

      a) Prevention of falling injury

      b) Elevate legs

      c) Loosen clothing around neck

      d) Wipe face with cool, wet cloth

      e) Seek medical attention if victim:

          1. Over the age of 40.

          2. Has repeated attacks.

          3. Looses consciousness while sitting and/or

          4. Faints with no apparent cause.

c. *Anaphylactic or Severe Allergic Shock* - Occurs when a previously sensitized person is exposed to an allergen, and the resulting antibody reaction triggers the release of chemical mediators such as histamine. This severe allergic response can be deadly due to swollen air passages and diminished circulation.

1) Signs and Symptoms include -

      a) Coughing, sneezing, and wheezing with dyspnea.

      b) Tightness in throat and chest.

      c) Severe itching, rash, or hives.

      d) Swelling of face, mouth, and tongue.
      e) Nausea and vomiting.
      f) Dizziness.
      g) Abdominal cramps.
      h) Cyanosis of lips and mouth.
      i) Unconsciousness.

  2) First Aid -
      a) Call 911 - This is a *true emergency*.
      b) Check **ABCs**.
      c) Administer epinephrine, using instructions if victim has anaphylaxis kit.

8. Bleeding and Wounds - Bleeding can be either internal and may not be visible or can be external which is visible. Rapid blood loss can lead to hypovolemic shock and must be treated immediately. Blood can be lost from arteries, veins, or capillaries. Blood loss from arteries is bright red and escapes with force. Blood loss from veins flows more slowly and is a darker red. Capillary leakage is usually slow and oozing.

  a. Signs and symptoms of bleeding include -
    1) Visual recognition of blood from skin or orifice.
    2) Bruises or contusions.
    3) Rapid pulse.
    4) Cold, moist skin.
    5) Dilated pupils.
    6) Nausea and vomiting.
    7) Bruised abdomen.
    8) Pain and bruising of chest.

  b. First Aid for Bleeding
    1) Locate bleeding source.
    2) Apply direct pressure to source.
    3) Elevate part above victim's heart.
    4) Apply pressure to "pressure point."
    5) Apply tourniquet.
    6) Treat for shock.
    7) Seek medical attention.

Wounds *may require stitches or professional medical attention if –*
    1) There is arterial or uncontrolled bleeding.
    2) Wounds show muscle or bony tissue, or gape widely.
    3) Wounds are large or deep (puncture).
    4) Wounds contain large or deeply embedded objects.
    5) Wounds are from animal or human bites.
    6) Wounds on areas that may leave conspicuous scars (face, etc).

Types of Open Wounds			
Type	**Cause**	**Signs/Symptoms**	**First Aid**
Abrasion (scrape)	Rubbing/scraping	Only skin surface affected Little bleeding	Remove all debris Wash with soap & water
Incision (Cut)	Sharp Objects	Smooth edges of wound. Severe bleeding	Control bleeding. Wash wound.
Laceration (Tear)	Blunt object	Veins/arteries can be affected - severe bleeding (danger of infection)	Control bleeding. Wash wound.
Puncture (stab)	Sharp/pointed object	Wound narrow/deep into veins/arteries; danger of infection	Do not remove impaled object
Avulsion (torn off)	Machinery, explosions	Tissue torn off/left hanging; severe bleeding	Control bleeding; take avulsed part to medical facility

9. Animal and Human Bites - Most bites do not cause significant bleeding, but are quite dangerous because of potential infection. 60-90% of all bites are from dogs. Human bites can cause serious injury, as they are more likely to become infected than bites from other warm blooded animals. Bites often require medical attention because they are difficult to thoroughly clean.

10. Specific Body Injuries -

a. Head, Neck, and Back Injuries -
1) *Skull Fracture* - Break or crack in the cranial bones. Presents with the following signs and symptoms:
a) Pain at the site of injury.
b) Deformity of skull or area of spine.
c) Bleeding from nose/ears.
d) Leaking of cerebral-spinal fluid.
e) Discoloration under eyes or behind the ear.
f) Unequal pupil size.
g) Profuse bleeding with exposure of skull or brain tissue.

2) *Concussion* - Change in brain function including loss of consciousness, resulting from a blow to the head. Signs and symptoms include:
a) Loss of consciousness.

b) Severe headache.

c) Amnesia.

d) Seeing stars.

e) Dizziness, weakness, double-vision.

Concussion Treatment Guidelines		
__Type__	__Description__	__Guidelines__
Mild	Momentary or no loss of consciousness.	Do not return to normal activities until medical evaluation made.
Moderate	Unconscious for less than five minutes.	Avoid vigorous activity for few days & resume only when associated symptoms have been resolved. Medical clearance.
Severe	Unconscious for more than than five minutes.	Avoid rigorous activity, for one month or longer; get neurologists clearance to return to normal activities.

3) *Contusions* - Caused by blows to the head but involve bruising and swelling of the brain. Lost blood may accumulate inside the skull and put pressure on the brain.

    a) Signs and symptoms include -

        1. Unconsciousness.

        2. Paralysis or weakness.

        3. Unequal pupil size/blurred vision.

        4. Vomiting and nausea.

        5. Amnesia.

        6. Headaches.

    b) *First Aid for Head, Neck and Back Injuries* -

        1. Maintain open airway.

        2. Minimize movement of head, neck & back.

        3. Control external bleeding.

        4. Check consciousness & breathing.

        5. Keep victim from getting chilled or overheated.

        6. Seek medical attention.

        7. Observe for signs and symptoms.

b. *Eye Injuries* - Require prompt attention by a medical professional because it is difficult to determine the extent of damage.

c. *Nose Bleeds* - Often self-limiting, yet produces anxiety in both victim and caregiver. Occasionally severe bleeding requires medical attention. Bleeding from a single nostril can often be stopped by applying pressure with the fingers to side of nose. Bleeding from the posterior part of the nose into the mouth and throat indicates a serious medical situation.

d. ***Dental and Oral Injuries*** - Require timely medical intervention. Seek medical assistance from a dentist or ER immediately.

e. *Abdominal Injuries* - Can be either open or closed, and may result in bleeding from damage to the abdominal wall or internal organs.

    1) Signs and symptoms include -
        a) Pain/cramping in abdomen.
        b) Legs drawn to chest.
        c) Nausea and vomiting.
        d) Skin wounds and penetrations.
        e) Protruding organs.
        f) Blood in urine or stool.
        g) Guarding of abdomen.
        h) Rapid pulse.
        i) Moist/cold skin.

    2) First Aid for Abdominal Injuries -
        a) Check ABCs and treat accordingly.
        b) Seek medical attention (*give no fluids or food*).

f. *Blister* - Results from excessive friction to the skin and is a collection of fluid between the layers of skin. Blisters are often accompanied by pain and redness in the immediate area. Blisters are usually self-limiting and should not be broken unless pain is unbearable because of possible infection. Use sterile technique and dressing if blister must be broken. Observe for signs of infection.

g. *Poisoning* - May result from ingesting toxins, insect or snakebites, exposure to allergic plants, or exposure to toxic gasses. The toxic substance damages tissue and can adversely affect organ system functioning. Poisonings are common among children, yet account for relatively few deaths among Americans. Swallowed poisons are the most commonly reported and many of these are treated by phone instructions. Insect stings are deadly for the allergic victim and require immediate intervention. Snakebites are seldom causes of death, with children being the most vulnerable victim. Seek medical attention immediately. Poisoning from plants is seldom life threatening but often severe. If symptoms are severe and persistent, seek medical advice. The possibility of inhaled poisons (such as carbon monoxide) can be difficult to evaluate, as many are odorless or tasteless. If symptoms exist, remove victim to a source of fresh air. Check ABCs and seek medical assistance.

h. *Burns* - More than two million burns occur each year leading to over 6,000 deaths in the U.S. Burns result from heat, UV light exposure, chemical exposure, or electrical shock.

Burn injuries range from mild to severe. Mild burns are known as first degree or superficial. They cause some minor discomfort and reddening of the skin. Moderate burns are known as second degree or partial thickness. They involve deep epidermal layers and are characterized by blisters, severe pain, generalized swelling, and fluid loss. Severe burns are known as third degree or full thickness, and are characterized by complete destruction of both the epidermis and dermis. Third degree burns may involve underlying muscle of bony tissue, and may temporarily present with less pain due to the destruction of nerve tissue. Fluid loss from third degree burns can be life threatening.

Burn injuries should also be assessed according to how much tissue is damaged, what parts of the body are burned, and how old the burn victim is. One method of estimating the amount of total skin surface involved is known as the "rule of nines". The body is divided into 11 areas of 9% each, with the area around the genitals representing an additional 1%. In the adult, 9% of the skin covers the head and each extremity (including both front & back). Twice as much, or 18%, of total skin area covers the front and back of the trunk and each lower extremity.

Severe second degree and all third degree burns need medical attention. Burns are classified accordingly, and considerations for assessment are included in the following table. Take into account the age of the victim, the classification of burn, and the amount of total skin surface burned.

First Aid for Burns		
Burn	**Do this**	**Don't do this**
1st degree (redness/mild swelling/pain)	Apply cold water and/or dry sterile dressing.	Apply ointments, butter, etc.
2nd degree (deeper; blisters)	Immerse cold water, blot dry with sterile cloth. Treat for shock Obtain medical attention.	Break blisters/ remove shreds of tissue. Use antiseptic/ointments etc.
3rd degree (deeper destruction/ skin layers destroyed)	Cover with sterile cloth. Treat for shock. Watch breathing & obtain immediate medical care.	Remove charred clothing. Apply ice. Use home medication.

i. *Cold Related Injuries* -

1) *Frostbite* occurs when the temperature of tissue drops below 32 degrees F. Damage occurs because of tissue "freezing" and the decrease in blood supply. Frostbite mainly affects the hands, feet, ears, and nose. All frostbite injuries require immediate attention.

2) *Hypothermia* results when the body's core temperature is reduced. A rectal or body temperature above 90 degrees F categorizes mild hypothermia. Symptoms include shivering, slurred speech, memory loss, and staggering gait. Most victims are conscious. Profound hypothermia will have a rectal or body temperature below 90 degrees F., with rigidity, blueness of skin, and unconsciousness. Either category requires medical intervention.

j. *Heat Related Injuries* - Include two major types (*heat stroke* and *heat exhaustion*) and two minor types (*heat cramps* and *heat syncope*, which resembles fainting & is usually self-limiting). The following charts describe heat related emergencies and their indicators:

Heat Related Emergencies			
Indicators:	*Heat Cramps (least serious)*	*Heat Exhaustion (serious)*	*Heat Stroke (most serious)*
Muscle cramps	Yes	No	No
Skin	Normal	Cold, clammy	Hot, dry
Temperature	Normal	Normal or slightly elevated	>105 degrees F.
Conscious	Usually	Sometimes	Usually unconscious
Perspiration	Heavy	Heavy	Little or none
First Aid	Move to cool area. Rest affected muscle. Give lots of water. **Do Not Massage.**	Move to cool area Elevate legs. Cool victim. If no improvement within 30 minutes, seek medical care.	Move to cool area. Elevate head/shoulder Cool victim. Transport for immediate medical care. Monitor ABCs. *Life threatening*!

k. *Bone, Joint, & Muscle Injuries -*

1) *Fractures* result when a bone is broken or cracked and are classified as either open (skin is broken) or closed.

    a) Signs and symptoms include -
        1. Swelling
        2. Deformity
        3. Pain/tenderness
        4. Loss of function
        5. Grating sensation or noise
        6. History of the injury

    b) First aid includes the control of bleeding (if present), splinting and calling for medical assistance.

2) *Spinal injuries* result commonly from auto/cycle accidents, falls, and diving accidents.

    a) Signs and symptoms include -
        1. History of injury
        2. Head injuries (15-20% also have spinal injuries)
        3. Painful movement of extremities
        4. Numbness, tingling, or burning sensation
        5. Loss of bowel/bladder control
        6. Paralysis
        7. Deformity

    b) Asking such questions as "Can you move your feet/fingers etc." gives clues to assessment. ***Any suspected spinal injury*** requires leaving the victim in their present position (unless danger persists), and waiting for trained assistance (EMS). Continue to monitor ABCs.

3) *Muscle* and *Joint Injuries* include *strains*, *sprains*, *contusions* and *cramps* (see pathology section for details)

First Aid for Strains and Sprains –
    R.I.C.E. (Rest, Ice, Compression, & Elevation) for *first 48-72 hours*. Serious injury to soft tissue requires immediate medical attention. RICE while awaiting medical care.

Business Practices, Professional Standards, Ethics, & First Aid /CPR
Review Questions

1. Which action demonstrates ethical standards & professionalism?
   a. Your client wants a reflexology session; you are not formally trained and refer your client to a reflexologist.
   b. Your client has a very emotional release during the massage; you continue the massage & attempt to counsel them.
   c. A client is visibly intoxicated & in a very boisterous mood; you try to calm them down & proceed with the massage, thinking they may relax.
   d. A wealthy client invites you and your family to use his beachfront condo for your two week vacation (you are currently doing insurance related massage work prescribed as a result of a car accident). You accept and thank him for his generosity.

2. Your client tells you he feels very faint. You should:
   a. Attempt to assist your client to a seat to prevent falling injuries.
   b. Elevate his legs.
   c. Loosen clothing around his neck.
   d. All of the above.

3. A marathon runner comes to you for massage after the race. The runner's skin is dry & hot; he is not perspiring, and feels faint. *Circle* the incorrect statement:
   a. It appears the runner is suffering from heat exhaustion.
   b. Elevate the head and shoulders.
   c. If possible move to cool area & attempt to cool victim.
   d. Summons medical attention immediately & monitor ABCs.

4. *Circle* the correct statement(s) regarding business practices:
   a. Barter income is not included in your total income for tax purposes since you received no money, but only exchanged services.
   b. A written contract is necessary if you are an independent contractor.
   c. Form W-2 is issued to independent contractors for income tax purposes.
   d. Income tax is withheld from income paid to an independent contractor.

5. A runner comes to the massage tent and complains of a sharp pain around her ankle. She twisted her ankle while running. She is limping and appears to have a deformity of the joint and hypermobility. The ankle is quite swollen. *Circle* the *incorrect* statement:
   a. Assist the runner to the medical tent for assistance.
   b. RICE is the appropriate protocol for the first 48-72 hours.
   c. It appears the runner has sustained a strain.
   d. It appears the runner has sustained a sprain.

6. The immediate First Aid actions required in treating an injured person are:
   a. Talk to the individual; determine if they are responsive.
   b. If possible, position the individual on their back (unless vomiting).
   c. Call 911 or other EMS giving exact location with identifying landmarks, your phone number, nature of the injury, condition of victim, what is being done, & any special circumstances.
   d. All of the above.

7. If you are a sole-proprietor, you are:
   a. Required to maintain complete records regarding income and expenses.
   b. Only required to pay your income & social security taxes when you file a tax return.
   c. Required to file a Schedule K-1 with your income tax return.
   d. All of the above.

8. You are presented with an athlete who just completed a marathon. His skin is cold & clammy, his temperature appears close to normal & he is perspiring very heavily. He may be suffering from:
   a. Heat cramps.
   b. Heat exhaustion.
   c. Heat stroke.
   d. Hypothermia.

9. You are self-employed. How often do you have to make estimated tax payments?
   a. Once a month.
   b. Annually, before December 31st of the tax year.
   c. You do not; just pay your taxes before April 15 when the return is due.
   d. Quarterly.

10. When administering first aid, your goal is to obtain all the necessary information related to the injury. You should conduct a primary survey of the situation, which includes:
    a. Checking the ABCs: airway, breathing, circulation, & hemorrhaging.
    b. Using universal precautions when administering *any* first aid.
    c. Assessing the victim's immediate condition & any unforeseen problems.
    d. All of the above.

11. You are a partner in a massage business. The partnership must:
    a. File Form 1065 annually.
    b. Issue a Schedule K-1 to each partner.
    c. Maintain all income and expense records. Claim all business expenses on Form 1065.
    d. All of the above.

12. *Circle* the correct statement:
   a. Malpractice insurance is required by law.
   b. Liability insurance and malpractice insurance are synonymous.
   c. LMT's are required to abide by all state and local regulations, which include the requirement for establishments to carry property damage and bodily injury liability insurance coverage.
   d. All of the above.

13. Your client arrives for his appointment & tells you he does not feel well. His lips are bluish; his skin is pale, cool, & clammy; pulse is rapid; he is breathing rapidly and feels nauseous. Circle the correct answer.
   a. Help him lie down on his side & try to keep him warm while you call EMS.
   b. Elevate his head & ask him to rest for a while. You'll check on him in a few minutes.
   c. It appears he may be suffering from anaphylactic shock.
   d. You reschedule the massage because he is not feeling well and send him home.

14. The client-therapist relationship is based on honest/open communication; this relationship includes:
   a. Maintaining client confidentiality.
   b. Educating the client regarding the benefits of massage.
   c. Respecting their pain tolerance, boundaries, and wishes.
   d. All of the above.

15. A runner comes to the massage tent seeking a massage because they are experiencing severe leg cramps. What is the appropriate action?
   a. Work the leg muscles with deep gliding strokes and apply direct pressure to the area of hyper constriction.
   b. Tell the client to "walk off the cramps" and then return for a massage.
   c. Stretch the leg muscles involved and massage the rest of their body.
   d. Assist if necessary, but refer to medical tent.

16. Your client has come in for neuromuscular work on an area of chronic pain, resulting from an auto accident. During your initial palpation the client keeps wincing. *Circle* the appropriate response:
   a. Explain to the client that your pressure is appropriate for the techniques you must use and that "no pain--no gain."
   b. Reluctantly lighten your pressure and explain that you will need to increase the pressure because it is necessary for an effective treatment.
   c. Immediately lighten your pressure and work within their pain tolerance.
   d. Apologize for hurting them and avoid the very sensitive areas.

17. Your client's chief complaint has been low back pain. This is their fifth visit and although they feel better for a day or two they are not making any substantial progress. Select the best response:
    a. Explain to them that it appears massage cannot help their condition.
    b. Refer them to your family physician.
    c. Explain to them that it sometimes takes many treatments to relieve chronic pain & that sometimes one may feel worse before beginning to feel better.
    d. Refer them to a M.D. (orthopedist) for an evaluation.

18. Universal precautions are used when administering First Aid because:
    Circle the correct statement(s):
    a. One has to assume that *anyone* receiving First Aid potentially has an infectious disease.
    b. HIV is transmitted by exposure to blood and other body fluids.
    c. Hepatitis & other pathogens are transmitted by exposure to blood & other body fluids.
    d. All of the above.

19. Confidentiality of your client's records is required for many reasons. The primary reason is:
    a. To protect yourself if sued by the client.
    b. To ensure adequate information for insurance billing purposes.
    c. Professional ethics.
    d. You were told to do so by your Swedish instructor.

20. If you find yourself in a situation where an individual requires First Aid:
    Circle the correct answer(s):
    a. You are only required to administer First Aid if you want to.
    b. If you acted in "good faith" & within the level of your training, you cannot be sued by an injured person.
    c. You must provide the level of care expected of a responsible person with the same training.
    d. All of the above.

VI   0ANSWER KEY

I.   Anatomy, Physiology, & Kinesiology

1.	a	31.	c	61.	d
2.	c	32.	d	62.	c
3.	d	33.	b	63.	b
4.	b	34.	d	64.	a
5.	b	35.	a	65.	a
6.	d	36.	d	66.	c
7.	a	37.	c	67.	d
8.	c	38.	d	68.	c
9.	d	39.	b	69.	d
10.	b	40.	c	70.	b
11.	d	41.	a	71.	c
12.	c	42.	d	72.	d
13.	a	43.	b	73.	b
14.	c	44.	d	74.	c
15.	d	45.	b	75.	b
16.	d	46.	b	76.	c
17.	c	47.	c	77.	c
18.	d	48.	d	78.	c
19.	a	49.	c	79.	a
20.	b	50.	d	80.	c
21.	d	51.	c	81.	b
22.	b	52.	a	82.	a
23.	c	53.	b	83.	a
24.	d	54.	b	84.	d
25.	a	55.	c	85.	c
26.	c	56.	d	86.	d
27.	c	57.	c	87.	b
28.	b	58.	a	88.	c
29.	a	59.	c	89.	a
30.	a	60.	a	90.	d

II.   Clinical Pathology

1.	b	10.	c	19.	a
2.	c	11.	b	20.	c
3.	b	12.	a	21.	b
4.	d	13.	c	22.	b
5.	d	14.	d	23.	b
6.	c	15.	c	24.	b
7.	d	16.	a	25.	a
8.	c	17.	c
9.	d	18.	b

III-A. Massage/Bodywork Theory, Assessment And Practice

1.	c	27.	c	53.	b
2.	c	28.	d	54.	d
3.	c	29.	d	55.	d
4.	b	30.	d	56.	d
5.	d	31.	d	57.	d
6.	d	32.	c	58.	b
7.	d	33.	d	59.	d
8.	a	34.	d	60.	b
9.	d	35.	b	61.	d
10.	b	36.	a	62.	d
11.	b	37.	d	63.	d
12.	b	38.	d	64.	c
13.	d	39.	d	65.	b
14.	c	40.	a	66.	a
15.	a	41.	d	67.	d
16.	a	42.	c	68.	d
17.	c	43.	d	69.	a
18.	c	44.	c	70.	b
19.	d	45.	a	71.	a
20.	c	46.	a	72.	d
21.	c	47.	b	73.	d
22.	a	48.	a	74.	d
23.	a	49.	c	75.	b
24.	c	50.	c	76.	c
25.	a	51.	d		
26.	a	52.	d		

III-B. Adjunct Techniques And Methods

1.	b	8.	d	15.	b
2.	c	9.	a	16.	d
3.	b	10.	d	17.	c
4.	b	11.	d	18.	c
5.	d	12.	d	19.	b
6.	c	13.	d	20.	c
7.	b	14.	b		

IV. Business Practices And Professionalism

1.	a	8.	b	15.	d
2.	d	9.	d	16.	c
3.	a	10.	d	17.	d
4.	b	11.	d	18.	d
5.	c	12.	c	19.	c
6.	d	13.	a	20.	c
7.	a	14.	d		

VII   WORKS CITED

American Red Cross. *Community First Aid and Safety*. San Bruno: StayWell, 2002.

Altug, Ziya, Janet Hoffman and Jerome Martin. *Manual of Clinical Exercise Testing, Prescription and Rehabilitation*. Norwalk: Appleton & Lange, 1993.

Ashley, Martin. *Massage, a Career At Your Fingertips*.3rd Edition. Carmel: Enterprise Publishing, 1999.

Barron, Patrick. *Hydrotherapy Theory & Technique*. 3rd Edition. St. James City: Pine Island Publishers, Inc., 2003.

Bates, Barbara. *A Guide to Physical Examination*. Philadelphia: J.B. Lippincott Co., 1974.

Beck, Mark. *The Theory and Practice of Therapeutic Massage*, Albany: Milady Publishing Corporation, 1988.

Beresford-Cooke, Carola. *Shiatsu Theory and Practice*. London: Churchill Livingston, 1996.

Cailliet, Rene. *Soft Tissue Pain and Disability*. 2nd Edition. Philadelphia: F.A. Davis Company, 1988.

Calais-Germain, Blandine. *Anatomy of Movement*. Seattle: Eastland Press, 1993.

Chengman, Sun. *Chinese Bodywork*. Berkeley: Pacific View Press, 1993.

Clarke, Sue. *Essential Chemistry for Safe Aromatherapy*. New York: Churchill Livingston, 2002.

Clemente, Carmine D. *Anatomy: A Regional Atlas of the Human Body*. 3rd Edition. Baltimore: Urban & Schwrzenberg, 1987.

Cotran, Ramzi, Vinay Kumar, and Tucker Collins. *Robbins Pathologic Basis of Disease.* 6th Edition. New York: Saunders, 2000.

Deadman, Peter and Al Khafaji, Mazin. *A Manual of Acupuncture*. East Sussex, England: Journal of Chinese Medical Publications, 1998.

Fritz, Sandy. *Mosby's Fundamentals of Therapeutic Mass*age. 2nd Edition. St. Louis: Mosby Inc., 2000.

Fritz, Sandy, Grosenbach, M James. *Essential Sciences for Therapeutic Massage*. St. Louis: Mosby, 2004.

Graham, Douglas. *Treatise on Massage, Its History, Mode of Application and Effects*.

Greenman, Phillip. *Principles of Manual Medicine*. 2nd Edition. Baltimore: Lippincott, Williams & Wilkins, 1996.

Hoppenfeld, Stanley. *Physical Examination of the Spine and Extremities*. New York: Appleton-Century-Crafts, 1976.

Juhan, Deane. *Job's Body-A Handbook for Bodywork*. Barrytown: Station Hill Press, 1987.

Kellogg, John Harvey. *The Art of Massage*. Montana: Kessinger Publishing Co., 1929.

Kendall, Florence, et al. *Muscles Testing and Function*. 3rd Edition. Baltimore: Williams & Wilkins, 1983

Kent, Thomas H. and Hart, Michael Noel. *Introduction to Human Disease*. East Norwalk: Appleton & Lange, 1993.

Kulund, Daniel N., M.D. *The Injured Athlete*. Philadelphia: J.B. Lippincott Co., 1988.

Lane, Keryn AG. *The Merck Manual*. 17th Edition. West Point: Merck & Co. 1999

Lowe, Whitney. *Functional Assessment in Massage Therapy*. 3rd Edition. Bend: OMERI, 1997.

Maciocia, Giovanni. *The Foundations of Chinese Medicine*. Edinburgh: Churchill Livingstone, 1998.

Magee, David, J. *Orthopedic Physical Assessment*. Philadelphia: W.B. Saunders, 1987.

Mao-Ling, Qiu. *Chinese Acupuncture & Moxibustion*. Shanghai: Shanghai Scientific & Technical Publications, 1996.

McCarty, Patrick. *Beginner's Guide to Shiatsu*. Eureka: Turning Point Publications, 1985.

Moor and Peterson, et al. *Manual of Hydrotherapy and Massage*. Mountain View: Pacific Press Publishing Assoc., 1964.

Moyers, Bill. *Healing and The Mind*. New York: Doubleday, 1995.

Peper, Erik Ph.D. Repetitive Strain Injury, *Physical Therapy Products*. Sept. 1994,

Reider, Bruce, MD. *The Orthopedic Physical Examination*. Philadelphia: W.B. Saunders Company, 1999.

Roy, Steven, and Richard Irvin. *Sports Medicine, Prevention, Evaluation, Management, and Rehabilitation*. St. Louis: Prentice Hall Publishing Inc., 1983.

Salvo, Susan G. *Massage Therapy Principles & Practice*. Philadelphia: W.B. Saunders Company, 1999.

Selye, Hans. *The Stress of Life*. New York: McGraw-Hill Book Co., 1956.

Sohn, Tina and Robert. *Amma Therapy*. Rochester, VT: Healing Arts Press, 1996.

Sohnen-Moe, Cherie M. *Business Mastery*. 3rd Edition. Tucson: Sohnen-Moe Associates, 1997.

Stein, Diane. *Essential Reiki: a complete guide to the ancient healing art*. Freedom: The Crossing Press, 1997.

Tappan, Frances M. and Patricia J. Benjamin. *Tappan's Healing Massage Techniques: Classic, Holistic, and Emerging Methods*. 4th Edition. Upper Saddle River: Pearson Education, Inc., 2005.

Thibodeau/Patton. *The Human Body in Health & Disease*. St. Louis: Mosby Year Book, 1992.

Thomas, C.L.; ed. *Taber's Cyclopedic Medical Dictionary*. 16th Edition. Philadelphia: F.A. Davis Co., 1989.

Thompson, Diana L. *Hands Heal*. 2nd Edition. Philadelphia: Lippincott Williams & Wilkins, 2002.

Thrash, Agatha and Calvin. *Home Remedies, Hydrotherapy, Massage, Charcoal & Other Simple Treatments*. Seale: Thrash Publications, 1981.

Tortora & Grabowski. *Principles Of Anatomy and Physiology*. 10th Edition. New York: John Wiley and Sons Inc., 2003.

Travell & Simons. *Myofascial Pain and Dysfunction: The Trigger Point Manual*. Volumes I & II. Philadelphia: William & Wilkins, 1992, 1995.

Xinnong, Cheng. *Chinese Acupuncture and Moxibustion*. Beijing: Foreign Language Press, 1990.

Yates, John. *A Physician's Guide to Therapeutic Massage*. Vancouver: Massage Therapists' Association of British Columbia, 1990.

VIII Index